HUSBAND'S GUIDE TO BREAST CANCER

A Complete & Concise Plan for Every Stage

Todd Outcalt

Blue River Press
Indianapolis

Husband's Guide to Breast Cancer © 2013 Todd Outcalt
Library of Congress Conotrol Number: 2013945326

Author photo on page 191 by Jeff Hayes
Cover designed by Heather Phillips, cover photo © RelaxFoto.de/iStockphoto
Packaged by Wish Publishing
Proofread by Dorothy Chambers
Index by AMI indexing

Printed in the United States of America
10 9 8 7 6 5 4 3 2 1

Distributed in the United States by
Cardinal Publishers Group
www.cardinalpub.com

Interior photos:
page 11 photo © Monkey Business Images/Shutterstock.com
page 44 photos: rose ©Elena Itsenko/Shutterstock.com, fruit ©Africa Studio/Shutterstock.com, pillows ©Africa Studio/Shutterstock.com, wedding photo©schemishev/Shutterstock.com, bath oils © Africa Studio/Shutterstock.com, frame©Liligraphie/Shutterstock.com
page 66 photos: hand©twobee/Shutterstock.com, wig©Sergey Goruppa/Shutterstock.com, husband and wife©Lisa F. Young/Shutterstock.com
page 94 photos: agent©Adam Gregor/Shutterstock.com, policy@S_L/Shutterstock.com, coins©Balefire/Shutterstock.com, coupons©trekandshoot/Shutterstock.com
pages 110-111 photos: oven cleaning ©Anne Kitzman/Shutterstock.com, husband and wife©Lisa F. Young/Shutterstock.com, vacuuming ©Tatyana Vyc/Shutterstock.com, grandma baking ©Mat Hayward/Shutterstock.com
pages 128-129 photos: vacation©Alan Bailey/Shutterstock.com, exercising©Monkey Business Images/Shutterstock.com, fundraiser©pics721/Shutterstock.com

The Explorer Turns Toward Home
—To Becky

I have sailed vast seas in search of you
And slogged through jungles dark with poison vine,
Charted the far lands of Timbuktu
While tortured by the fly and porcupine.
I have dodged pits and hungry cannibals,
Persevered through sleet and spitting snow,
Oared down rivers, survived waterfalls
And mutinous friends who craved the status-quo.
And I have seen the end of earth and time:
Unknown cultures, forests, desert plains,
Azure cities, mountains I could not climb,
Such beauties now but where your heart remains.
But as I turn toward home my sustenance
Is you, and I desire your face above these continents.

Table of Contents

Acknowledgments

I have always viewed book writing as a great gift, and as far as bringing a book into existence, a debt of gratitude must be extended to the many who make it possible. First, I wish to thank Tom Doherty for serving as publisher, guide and visionary—and all the staff at the Cardinal Group, including Holly Kondras for her editorial recommendations and insights for strengthening the whole. Books don't just happen ... they are created.

I also thank my wife, Becky, for agreeing to open our lives and history to others. She is certainly the inspiration behind this book and continues to show me, day by day, how a person can re-create a life after breast cancer. During our more-than-thirty years of marriage, we have also had the opportunity to help other couples, and we hope this book will be another brick in that wall of encouragement. Although a breast cancer history is only a small portion of our marriage, I am thankful that my wife doesn't just define herself as "breast cancer survivor," but also as wife, mother, friend and colleague. Becky continues to inspire me daily, and I want this book to say "I love you."

There are dozens of men and women who have shared their breast cancer experiences with me through the years, and I thank everyone who made themselves available for my incessant questions, interviews and follow-up phone conversations. Whether mentioned by name in this book or not, in one way or another I have learned something from every man who was bold enough to share his thoughts, feelings and experiences about the breast cancer battle. And I am particularly grateful to those men (and couples) who agreed to share their stories in much richer detail for a general audience. Some of your names, at your request, have been changed for these pages, but you know who you are, and I thank you for being a part of this book.

I am also grateful to the various editors who have published my past articles and essays about breast cancer (even some poems), and I would here like to recognize the staff at magazines like

Cure, The Way of St. Francis, and *The Barefoot Review* for their support and encouragement through the years. Thank you for giving me a forum for sharing a narrative or two, or maybe some insights, about the breast cancer journey.

Additionally, I have to thank my daughter, Chelsey, and my son, Logan, for their strong attitudes and resiliency through the years, and for supporting my writing endeavors their entire lifetimes. Both of you are strong writers yourselves, and I hope you will find the outlets for your own creative vision in the years ahead.

I must thank the congregations I have served. First, at University Heights—for the kindnesses and support extended during Becky's months of healing and for providing that first line of defense when a family is faced with the brutal realities of breast cancer. I also thank Calvary United Methodist Church in Brownsburg—for always showing me incredible support and friendship while I serve as your pastor, and also for encouraging me to keep writing in the wee hours of the morning and late into the night. And thank you to those friends from both congregations who have shared more deeply in the breast cancer journeys they have experienced and made portions of this book possible through their testimonies.

And, although not directly related to this book, I would like to thank the Lilly Foundation for providing a sabbatical in 2002 that enabled me to conduct breast cancer research, write *The Healing Touch* (HCI), and refresh my spirit so that I could be far more effective as a husband, father, pastor and friend. The spirit of that refreshment is part and parcel of this book, and I thank the Lilly Endowment for making it possible.

For the many books I have read over the years, I would also like to thank those authors who have added to my knowledge of breast cancer, or created a greater awareness of what healing can look like, or even brightened my hope for impacting those women and the men who help others through illness. I do appreciate the research and knowledge gleaned, and trust that this book can add not only to the conversation but also to the hope for a cure.

My thanks also goes out to Rob Probus at Beacon Bulb for producing my CD, *Caring Through Cancer: A Caregiver's Guide*. Some bits and pieces of this CD are incorporated into the mix of this book, and I'm grateful to have added an audio aid to the conversation. Thanks, Rob, for your excellence in all aspects of that production.

And finally, I wish to thank the readers who, hopefully, will find encouragement and support through these pages. Any deficiencies are mine, and I hope you can look beyond them to continue your pursuit of healing and support in your own breast cancer journeys.

Husband's Quick Guide
Top 10 Things to Remember

In the event you are not a reader, or you feel that you don't have the time or energy to peruse this entire book, here are the top 10 things to remember from diagnosis, to prognosis, to the treatment, and beyond. Keep this guide handy and refer to it often.

1. Remember: A breast cancer diagnosis is not a death sentence. Remind your wife often that she will be a cancer survivor. Most breast cancer diagnoses are not emergencies, and breast cancer is highly treatable.

2. Do your research on breast cancer, understand the treatments available, and gather your support team (doctors, family, friends) to help your wife in her journey toward healing.

3. In all things remember: be there for her. When in doubt, be a man and do more.

4. Your family—even younger children—can be a source of strength, encouragement and inspiration to your wife.

5. As the husband, be prepared to do the hard work of following up with your insurance company, clarifying coverage, and when necessary, working out a payment plan for the cost of care.

6. Listen closely, take notes, and work hard at understanding your wife's breast cancer and what will be required for her treatment. This may or may not include a lumpectomy or mastectomy, radiation therapy, chemotherapy, reconstruction surgery, and follow-up surgery.

7. The road to your wife's recovery may include time off after surgery and therapy (radiation or chemo). This recovery period will be when you will lend your greatest support—with your time and attention, your love, your parenting, and your help around the house.

8. As the months and years go by following your wife's recovery, you will have many milestones to celebrate. In some ways you will be building a new life, post-cancer, and this may include certain changes in your lifestyle, diet, exercise, sexuality and priorities.

9. If your wife develops difficulties such as lymphedema or needs hormone replacement therapy, these can be treated or managed.

10. If your wife is in that small percentage of women who develops a metastatic form of cancer, there is much support available to help her, and you, through all of these advanced stages of the disease.

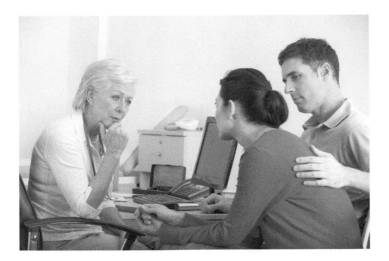

Foreword

During the years leading up to the writing of this book, I was blessed to be able to talk to dozens of women and men who were willing to share insights about their breast cancer journeys. I have learned something from every one of them.

In the process of writing this book, I also interviewed other couples (and men) who were willing to share bits and pieces of their own experiences. Some of these experiences have been incorporated into this book in the form of first person narratives in each chapter, and the quotes provided are also from many of these conversations. Some names have been changed in order to protect the privacy of friends, but the narratives are true-life stories filled with the anxiety, stresses, hopes, and healings that others wished to tell. In many respects, these narratives are the backbone of the book, as I have always felt that we can learn much from listening to others and gleaning the benefit of past experiences.

Again, I want to thank the couples (men and women alike) who were willing to tell me their stories and answer my questions.

Likewise, I wanted to provide a helpful glossary of terms in the back of the book and a core bibliography that could provide suggestions for further reading. A list of top Web sites can also be found in the back, and the resources these provide are invaluable. Men should not let their research end with this book but continue to learn through some of these excellent books and options.

A list of breast cancer agencies and non-profit breast cancer institutions round out the book, and I hope readers will find the contact information helpful and inviting for further research and answers.

Finally, it is important to note that throughout this book, I will generally discuss the breast cancer journey in terms of "husbands and wives," but I realize this is not always the case among those who are reading the book. Some men may be helping their sisters, their mothers, their aunts, their girlfriends, or even a co-worker. And so while using the term "wife," I hope every man may be able to substitute for thier own relationship as they need to. I hope to be as inclusive as possible while also allowing the book to read smoothly.

So men, regardless of the relationship, the essential ingredient here is your care and your caregiving. That's why you are reading this ... and it's why I am writing for you. Thanks.

Introduction
Initial Reactions to Breast Cancer

As you begin this journey of being a support partner, it is of foremost importance to understand how a woman feels when she receives a breast cancer diagnosis (we'll get to *your* feelings later). After all, you will want to consider her feelings first—and it is vital that you try to understand her position.

Having talked with many breast cancer survivors over the years, there seem to be some common themes. And many doctors will also affirm them.

A woman's first reaction to receiving a breast cancer diagnosis usually comes in the form of a question: "Will I die?" And almost immediately thereafter she wonders: "Will I lose my breast(s)?" These questions are to be expected, and they come from a deep place where a woman begins to come to grips with her vulnerability—and then wonders about her body. What will happen to me? What is in store for me? What does this mean? These are the questions that can scroll through a woman's mind in those first minutes or hours.

Some women, especially younger women, can be shocked by the news that they have breast cancer. Even after a suspicious-looking mammogram or a biopsy, many younger women, especially, are unable to bring themselves to believe that cancer has invaded their bodies. This too, however, is understandable. (Men, for example, would be shocked to receive news that they have prostate cancer.)

The news can also be shocking to women because, in most cases, their bodies have not given them any advanced warning. Few women, for example, notice a lump in the breast during a self-exam. And very few women go to a mammogram appointment suspecting that something is awry inside their bodies. Few experience any pain, discomfort or symptoms related to breast cancer.

Likewise, most women also travel through the various stages of grief as they begin to cope with their diagnosis and learn more about it. Many women become angry. They cannot necessarily name this anger, and sometimes it may be released in the form of anger toward a spouse, or children, or even the doctors. Other women simply need to throw things or yell as a form of release. But this anger can also emerge because women feel that their bodies have somehow betrayed them or not functioned properly. Other women may even be angry at themselves at some point, wondering whether they ate the wrong foods, engaged in bad habits, or did something that caused their bodies to manufacture a cancer cell. None of these feelings, however, have any bearing on the breast cancer itself and rarely serve as an explanation for why cancer has formed in her breast. Some women will even continue to ask these questions for weeks as if trying to figure out a puzzle they cannot solve. And, of course, they won't solve it.

Frustration can set in. Confusion. And after this initial shock, many women are able to later express that these first hours/days were the worst part of the journey. As they begin to learn more about breast cancer, as they begin to ask questions and receive answers from the doctors, most women settle in with a resolve to battle the cancer and to make an informed decision regarding surgery and/or treatment.

One of my wife's friends, who is also a breast cancer survivor, expressed her initial reactions and feelings this way:

Of course I was in shock, but then my first thought was, "I want this out of my body!" All I could think about in those initial hours was having my breast removed. I even considered having both breasts removed although cancer had been detected only in one breast. I felt like my body had betrayed me and all I could think about was getting the disease removed. It took some days and follow-up conversations and assurances by the medical staff to convince me that I could fight the cancer without such a drastic response. I had to calm down before I could see things clearly and think about my options. I was glad the doctors didn't jump on my paranoia. They were patient, kind, very professional. They had seen this before, I'm sure. But I figured out my options once I had all the information and could find my balance again.

So ... every woman is different in response and approach, but as the caregiver, being aware of a woman's thoughts and feelings is paramount to helping. Be aware that your wife (or girlfriend , mother or sister) may have any of the aforementioned thoughts and feelings—but she may have others, too.

For example, some women may doubt their attractiveness or wonder if having a breast removed or augmented will affect their marriage. Others may wonder how breast cancer will impact their sex life or impact their sex appeal. Or, if their marriage is already strained or if there are questions about the future of the marriage, some women might pull closer to their husbands *or* distance themselves even further emotionally and physically.

But don't be afraid to express your own feelings, especially your love and support. Many men fear they will say "the wrong thing".

Some men, for example, might try to make things better by saying, "It's you I love, not your breasts." This can be comforting to some wives but might infuriate others. Other men might try to steer a positive course through these initial conversations—and there's nothing wrong with that—but not all women will respond well to uplifting thoughts (especially in the first days following a diagnosis). A positive spin on breast cancer might make a woman feel the disease is nothing to worry about, or it might actually make her feel even more vulnerable and lonely. Recognizing her feelings is never a bad place to begin.

A great place to start any conversation is "I know I don't understand everything you are feeling right now, but I want you to know I love you." Expressing this kind of support and empathy can never be a bad thing , but men shouldn't beat themselves up if they are doing the best they can and trying to show support.

Be kind to yourself and your wife in these beginning stages.

A man will need to be aware that a breast cancer diagnosis impacts more than just a woman's body. The diagnosis also impacts the marriage and the entire family dynamic. And if a man needs more help understanding this, he could consider how he might feel if he had to have surgery on his testicles or his penis. A woman's breasts can be far more representative of her sexuality and individuality than men realize, and caregiving can begin with this understanding and connection.

Although it is not always the case, many men also discover that a wife's breast cancer diagnosis is an opportunity for them to connect more deeply. Sometimes marriage can be strengthened through adversity—and breast cancer is all of that. Uncertainty and fear can also be a uniting force in a marriage, and many couples connect more strongly through the breast cancer journey, emerging on the other side of the healing with a much deeper love and respect for each other.

What Does Losing a Breast Mean?

Eventually a woman will ask the question: "What does losing this breast mean to me?" Women opting for mastectomies, especially, will need to come to grips with this one. Her answer(s) may be philosophical (it is only tissue), or medical (no more cancer in my body), or even deeply personal (I feel like I am losing a part of myself). Regardless, a man can play a large role in helping a woman feel loved and appreciated. Although she may be losing a breast, she is not alone in the journey.

Losing a breast, however, will impact a woman deeply. Some women may try to shove their feelings aside or pretend that losing a breast is unimportant, but deep down there may be questions. Some women may feel that they are no longer a "complete woman" or that, somehow, their feminine identity has been diminished. Other women may lose some of their self-confidence, or may feel the impact of the lost breast in their work, or position, or ability to lead. Our bodies are complex things—and we don't often realize how the loss of an organ can impact us on emotional and relational levels. The loss of a breast can also impact a woman's sexuality and desires.

Every woman has thoughts and feelings about her breasts. Even if she doesn't like her breasts especially, having one surgically removed can be a powerful event in her life. She may lean more heavily upon you during subsequent moments of uncertainty, and you can be there to pick her up and reassure her.

18

One comment that I recall from my wife's surgeon was this: the majority of women are more concerned with saving the breast than saving their own lives. Wow! That one shocked me. But in retrospect, I know it is true. My wife and I spent hours trying to figure out a "cure" that would not include a mastectomy. At one point, I recall that my wife even considered doing nothing—waiting to see if the cancer would disappear. It took several days for her (and me) to arrive at the conclusion that a mastectomy was the only viable option.

This is not true of every breast cancer diagnosis, of course. Your wife may, indeed, have other options and may not have to answer the question: "What does losing a breast mean to me?" But if she is forced to answer the question, you can be most helpful by giving her the space and the "permission" to let go. Naturally, you will be depending heavily upon your surgeon's recommendations at this point, but at the relational and emotional level, your support will be important.

Now ... What Are *You* Feeling?

Now that you understand your wife's feelings, let's discuss your emotions. Let's face it, a man may have a different slant or approach to a breast cancer diagnosis.

First, the fact that the breast cancer is not *your* cancer is a huge differentiation. Your wife may feel alone at times, but you may not understand all that she is going through as well. You are not your wife. You are not the one with cancer. She is the one with the disease, not you. So initially you may feel some distance from the diagnosis. It may seem surreal. You may think you misheard. You may think your wife is mistaken. This too shall pass ... .

You may also feel isolated.

Early on in my wife's journey, I recall feeling alone myself. I knew that other men—other husbands—had been through this, too, but I didn't know where to find them or how to approach the subject. I kept a great deal of my fear inside. Eventually I began writing down some of my thoughts, which helped immensely. But much of my trepidation was solitary. I bottled

19

up. I lost sleep. At first I didn't want to talk about the breast cancer and the choices my wife would have to make.

But this, too, I learned is normal.

Other men may initially react to a breast cancer diagnosis by dismissing it entirely. "Oh, this will pass," some might think. Or "this is a mistake, and we can correct it through a second opinion." Other men might even ask their wives to take a second test or consider standing pat and waiting to see what happens. Again, these are not unusual reactions from men. You may find yourself at just such a place.

Men also have a tendency to trend to the positive, so much so that many women aren't able to fully grieve or express their concerns or anxieties properly. For example, it really doesn't help for a man to say things like, "Everything will be okay ... don't worry about this" or "This will all work out just fine ... you'll see." A man may feel this way, but expressing these ideas on the tail end of the diagnosis simply glosses over the severity of breast cancer and is not helpful to a woman. Your positive energy and humor can help, but is best served later in the journey.

These are not the only feelings, however.

Most men also experience some form of anger. This anger may manifest itself as venting to your wife or quietly seething. You might be angry over the inconvenience of this disease or the fact that your wife has breast cancer or that breast cancer will be a hardship on the family. You may also be angry at your wife or fight back feelings of betrayal. You may feel that you didn't discuss this disease or factor it into your marriage plans or your life's goals. Although a man wouldn't blame his wife for having cancer, he might secretly be concerned about himself and wonder, "What did I do to deserve this?" It may take time to develop a healthy attitude toward the disease and the treatment.

But regardless of the source, be aware that anger may be a part of the equation initially. However, as you learn more about breast cancer and discuss prognosis and treatment with your wife, anger will fade and be replaced by deep concern. This initial anger can fuel your reservoir of energy and propel you to a new understanding.

Finally, men can also have deep-seated questions about a wife's breast cancer. Initially, or somewhere in the journey, a man may wonder, "How will my wife's appearance be affected if she loses a breast?" Many men don't express this concern openly, however, as it can seem selfish or superficial. We often keep these thoughts to ourselves, but we still wonder about them.

Many men don't express these concerns, openly, however, as these questions can seem selfish or superficial. We often keep these thoughts to ourselves—but we still wonder about them.

I know that soon after my wife decided to have her mastectomy, I began wondering about her appearance. I wasn't concerned about my reaction, however, but about her self-image and how others might regard her. Yes, I did wonder what a post-mastectomy breast looked like (before the breast implant), but I knew this would not weaken my attraction to my wife or my love for her. For me, it wasn't a worry about sexual attraction; it was a curiosity.

Nevertheless, in the weeks leading up to my wife's surgery, I recall having an infatuation with breasts. I spent a great deal of time thumbing through books that the surgeon had given us—photographic plates of women who had undergone radical mastectomies or breast reconstruction or who had breast implants inserted. I surfed the Internet in search of other mastectomy images and wondered how my wife's body would look in comparison to some of the post-surgical images I found online. For a few days, breasts were all I could think about.

Days later, when we met with the plastic surgeon, I recall his humor as he told me that I might want to "test run" some of the breast implants (for size, weight, feel) and that he could even give my wife a "size increase" if she wanted more to show. I laughed at his jokes, but inside I continued to wonder how all of this was impacting my wife and what her real desires were. I didn't want her to make a decision based on my opinion or preferences. In actuality, nothing mattered except her health and recovery, and I made certain she felt complete freedom in selecting her implant.

However, speaking to the plastic surgeon about the breast reconstruction was, in fact, one of the more challenging times for me. I continued to wonder what the final "appearance" would be, not because I thought I would find my wife less attractive, but because it was new territory for us both. I wanted my wife to be healthy and whole—and also feel good about her decision. And I wanted her to have a healthy self-esteem, too. This is something we actually talked about in detail: what the breast implant would be like, how the nipple would be reconstructed, when the nipple would be "tattooed." I had never considered all of the steps in the implant and image recovery, but it was all part of the journey.

Beyond the questions about the mastectomy and breast implant, I was also wondering about our sex life. So was my wife. Her concerns, I learned, were actually more pronounced than mine. She continued to wonder how the loss of a breast would impact her as a woman. I was more concerned with hurting her, especially in the early months following the surgery. Would I touch her in the wrong way? What if I accidently pressed too hard on her chest? Would she want me to touch her?

I had all of these questions and more.

But, like the post-surgical scar itself, all of these concerns eventually faded as we learned how to make love post-mastectomy, and in time there was no difference in our love-making at all. (Though, I must say, it's just gotten better through the years!) In fact, I discovered that my wife's reconstructed breast was not even a consideration. Most days, I didn't even think of my wife as a breast cancer survivor. And now—more than ten years later—I don't even notice anything about my wife's body that is related to the mastectomy scar or the implant. I just don't think about it. I just see *her*.

Time *and work* really do heal wounds.

I share these personal thoughts here because I know that most men have similar concerns early in the journey. But there is nothing to fear. With solid communication and deep love and respect, all things can heal.

All of these feelings are important, however, and men should not shy away from them. Even if you don't have an ability to express some of these feelings to your wife, you may have some trusted friends you could talk to, or you could always seek out other men whose wives have survived breast cancer. Believe me, there is a very large network for breast cancer out there. If you need a support group or even a short-term network of helpers, it is there.

A breast cancer husband will always remember the day his wife informed him of her breast cancer diagnosis. He can recall where he was and what he was doing. He may recall his initial thoughts and feelings. And if he is honest, he will also wonder about his ability to handle the crisis.

But while that day is unforgettable, the weeks and months following may be little more than a blur of activity and decisions. Most men will discover that, while they can help their wives process information, keep track of appointments, and make certain decisions regarding surgery and treatment, they wish there was information more specifically designed for them. If only they knew more. And they wish they could get at it quickly.

That's what I've attempted to do with this book: create a practical and straightforward guide that will provide men with the information they want . . . and at a glance. Tips, first-person accounts, bullet-point lists: a kind of pocketbook.

This book is not, however, meant to be a medical guide or a resource for making medical decisions. All medical guidance will need to come from your doctors, as this book is meant to provide only basic information about breast cancer, treatment, and caregiving. Hopefully, this book will contain some good questions, but the answers will come in your time and in your discussions with the doctors.

There are some wonderful first-person narratives here in this book and a great deal of pertinent information that should prove helpful. And there are far more resources listed in the back. The most important resource, however, is your care. The more of that you provide, the higher your stock rises.

You can help write this guide—*your guide*—to breast cancer.

Chapter One
Your Initial Conversations

In the days immediately following the breast cancer diagnosis, it is important to remember that everyone processes shock, sadness, anxiety, fear and anger in different ways and at different paces. You may discover, for example, that your wife is not eager to discuss her breast cancer right away, whereas you are anxious to work through all the information and make a decision. Or, it could be quite the opposite.

But no matter how different or similar you are in your pace and approach, it will be important for you to begin discussing the diagnosis and what it means. In the meantime, there are some non-threatening questions you can initiate that can open up the channels of communication.

For example, here are some helpful conversation starters that might set you on a path toward better understanding and common goals.

- I'm listening . . . can you tell me how you are feeling right now?

- What is the most helpful thing I can do for you right now?

- What fears do you have?

- What can I do to make this journey easier for you?

- What do you need from me in the coming weeks?

Your initial conversations about the diagnosis do not have to be decisive ones. You are not making decisions at this point but processing emotions and questions. Be patient. Be patient with each other.

You may discover that your initial conversations about breast cancer have little to do with cancer itself. Some of your concerns may center on family or children (more on this in Chapter Five). Other concerns may be financial (see Chapter Six). And still other concerns may relate to your work or trying to figure out schedules and conflicts in the coming weeks.

Again, every couple deals with a diagnosis differently, but you can rest assured that as you begin the journey together many of your conversations will become natural. You will think of questions you need to ask (write these down), or you might even relegate an entire evening or weekend to reading, researching and processing information. You will begin talking about your anxieties and hopes more openly, and eventually you will help your wife reach a decision that is right for her. And you will have been an integral part of the process.

Many couples also bring other family members and friends into the conversation (they can be supportive, too). Parents, brother and sisters, and even good friends can all add something to the journey—if they are willing and invited. But don't allow negativity or too many opinions to cloud the water, either.

These initial conversations you will have about breast cancer may be fraught with a great deal of emotion—hers *and yours*. In the initial hours or even days, you may discover that your wife oscillates between anger and depression, acceptance and shock, her old self and some new version of your wife that is now shot through with a strange mixture of strength and weakness. Keep in mind that your role won't be to answer all of her questions or to provide answers or solutions, or even to fix the problem for her. You couldn't do these things even if you wanted to. Rather, your initial conversations should focus on listening, showing your genuine care, and making certain she knows you are beside her and will support her in her fight.

Don't feel you have to do the talking. Let her speak. Or if she is asking your opinion, offer it with a caveat of "these are my feelings" or "I'm here to support what you decide."

No doubt these first conversations will seem odd to the both of you. In fact, you may discover that your discussions are opening up a whole new side to your relationship, deepening your love, or even exposing some past hurts. But think of these initial conversations as a way to strengthen your marriage, too. It can happen—it does to many couples.

And best of all—be yourself. Don't put on an act or try to become a doctor or a lawyer or someone you are not. Be the man she married. Be a good listener. And if you can do these things, you'll be a hero.

෨෬

First Person

I suppose my first thought was, "My wife's going to die." But then I realized that I knew a lot of women who were breast cancer survivors. I also knew we didn't know a whole lot about my wife's situation either. We had not met with a doctor. All we knew was that my wife had breast cancer.

The days in between the biopsy report and the first meeting with the doctor were not easy ones. We didn't sleep much. My wife didn't want to tell our kids anything until she knew more, so she kept the secret, which was difficult. We started reading about breast cancer and studying up on it, but I'm not sure that helped much at that point because we were reading about some frightening situations.

I know my wife felt alone at that time, and I really didn't know what to say or how to respond. In some ways we just wanted to get some answers—you know, find out exactly what my wife would be facing and what we would have to do to combat the cancer. I think we stayed up a couple of nights kind of late, just sitting together and wondering what would happen.

I do think that getting answers is a big relief—making a decision. Once you get past the initial shock and begin making a plan with the doctors, it all sort of falls into place and you have something to talk about. I'm a coach, and I felt like at that point I had a game plan. My wife felt the same way. She was relieved when she found out the cancer was in the very early stages, and she could probably just have a mastectomy and not have to worry about any radiation or chemo. There was no indication of cancer in her lymph nodes, so that was a big relief.

We feel very fortunate. A lot of women, I know, have to endure more.

27

It will sound trite, but I'd tell men not to worry until they have answers. That's easier said than done, I know. But I spent a lot of time running through scenarios in my head that, in fact, were not anything close to reality. I was just imagining the worst. I could have saved myself a lot of lost sleep if I'd just waited until after we talked to the doctors.

Then I'd worry (laughs).

I learned that my wife was a lot stronger than I gave her credit for. And she continues to surprise me. Now she's helping other women get through their ordeal. She's very involved in all of this from a supportive standpoint. I think she has walked for breast cancer, helped raise money and awareness, and she's even given a couple of talks at church about it. She's become a kind of expert, and a lot of women look to her for answers. I really admire that about her.

I was just glad I could be there for her. I'm not sure I did anything special that any other husband wouldn't do, but life is good.

~Ian

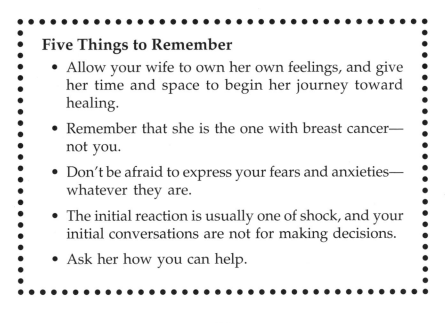

Five Things to Remember

- Allow your wife to own her own feelings, and give her time and space to begin her journey toward healing.

- Remember that she is the one with breast cancer— not you.

- Don't be afraid to express your fears and anxieties— whatever they are.

- The initial reaction is usually one of shock, and your initial conversations are not for making decisions.

- Ask her how you can help.

Chapter Two
What Does She Need?

Men are problem solvers. We are hot-wired for repair.

But even when we have no skills for problem solving, we tend to believe that we can fix a leaky sink, patch a hole in the wall, or repair a crack in the ceiling. We are problem solvers at work, too: writing reports, repairing an engine, or managing a large, eclectic staff of personalities. When there are problems, we go to work on finding a solution. Because of this tendency, it is our nature to believe that we have the skills necessary to deal with life's unexpected difficulties, too. Most men approach a problem by analyzing it, searching for weak points or loopholes, and then planning a point of attack.

But breast cancer is different. This is not a problem we will be able to fix. Certainly not by ourselves. And certainly not for the woman we love.

Nevertheless, most men try to approach a breast cancer diagnosis by using intellect—at least initially. We tend to believe that all a woman needs is the proper information, the right doctor, the best hospital, the perfect treatment. Problem solved.

Women, however, see things differently than men do.

In his classic couples book, *Men Are From Mars, Women Are From Venus,* John Gray outlines the differences between the sexes and the various ways men can be aware of a woman's needs. Although Gray's book doesn't address illness, there is much to be gleaned there when it comes to understanding the kind of emotional and relational support women desire.

While men are problem solvers and lone rangers, women tend more toward the relational spectrum of solutions, and they are looking for support as much as answers. Often, when a woman is expressing a problem at work or discussing a difficult day in the office, she is not looking for the man to provide an answer. She is, however, looking for a listening ear and a supportive presence. Holding a woman when she is frustrated can be much more soothing and supportive (from her perspective) than trying to trouble-shoot at the dinner table.

So when it comes to a breast cancer diagnosis, women aren't necessarily looking for a problem solver so much as a problem helper. My own experiences with couples bear this out in a myriad of ways.

Not long ago I was talking to a couple who had been going through a particularly rocky period in their marriage. The wife was expressing how distant her husband seemed and said he was unavailable to her. When I asked her to explain further, I learned that she had been diagnosed with breast cancer about eighteen months prior. This was when the marriage began to experience struggles.

"I didn't know what to do," the husband explained. "I tried my best to fix the problem, but she didn't seem interested in my advice."

"I wasn't looking for advice," the wife explained. "All I wanted was your presence and support. But you weren't there for me."

This type of scene, I'm afraid, can be lived out in many marriages, especially when an illness creates a new paradigm for marriage and men are thrown into situations that require their intellectual and emotional focus. Sometimes men can miss the mark. They mean well, but they don't understand what their wives (or mothers, sisters or girlfriends) really need.

When a woman has received a breast cancer diagnosis, she craves support and love more than anything else. She does not expect her husband (or brother, father or boyfriend) to swoop in and fix the problem. Rather, she *does* desire a man's help, but is looking for the emotional and physical strength a man can provide. Men cannot overlook this need. And there are hundreds of ways a man can provide this show of support.

Men can live up to this challenge. There are many practical ways men can demonstrate their care. All it takes is focus and commitment. And if a man is attentive, he can learn how to be the caregiver his wife needs.

Presence With a Purpose

As soon as a woman learns she has breast cancer, she is going to be engaged in a number of follow-up meetings with doctors, surgeons, nurses, and maybe even plastic surgeons, nutritionists and therapists. This may become a very time-consuming endeavor and also physically exhausting. And that's why one of the most important steps a man can take is to be aware that his presence will be her strong arm of support.

When my wife was going through her breast cancer conversations with doctors, I was amazed at the lack of support many women seemed to have. Often I would witness women emerging from these medical offices in tears, with no man nearby for comfort. In fact, it seemed that many of these women were going through the breast cancer journey alone. They appeared to be downcast—hopeless. I kept wondering: *Where are the men*?

The women who were accompanied by a man, however, seemed upbeat and strong. There was a determination in their faces, a kind of confidence. It was obvious when a woman had the support of a man, and I was always uplifted myself when I could talk to another guy in the waiting room or post-doctor visit.

I recall that, after sitting in on these long and arduous meetings with my wife, she would say to me later, "Thanks for going to this appointment with me." But my presence meant a great deal more. We became very close through the ordeal, and I actually looked forward to finding out from the doctors and surgeons what my role would be—what I could do to help my wife through the healing process. There was always something to do. I couldn't fix the problem for her, but there was never any lack of job security. I was motivated to work.

That's why you should never feel that your role is unimportant. Even to the doctors, your presence means a great deal, and doctors, I know, always appreciate a supportive cast when they are having a conversation about treatment options, surgical procedures, and even therapeutic exercises following surgery. Every woman needs someone to lean on. And a man's presence is crucial. You might even remember points from these conversations that your wife might overlook. As they say, "Two minds work better than one." Your wife may be distracted through portions of these medical conversations, so you can be the listener and the learner.

Most importantly, be present when your wife needs you. Find a way to rearrange your calendar. Create space for conversations with her. She will need time to mentally process her options, and she may use you as a sounding board. Again, you don't have to fix the problem—she doesn't expect you to. But you can be a good ear and show lots of empathy and understanding. You can ask good questions. You can help her to remember details of the conversations she had with doctors. Or you can also read some of the same material she is reading and offer your insights about what you are learning.

While your wife is waiting for her surgery or treatment, you may also discover new ways to spend time together. Go out to lunch together before or after her appointments. Take a walk. Sit in the park. Make time to be present. These times could mean more to her than you realize. Having these breaks together will not be making light of the cancer, and it will deepen your relationship.

After your wife's surgery or treatments, you will also need to be present in special ways: perhaps in those first few days, you will need to help change surgical dressings, or you may have to help your wife in and out of the shower, or even to the bathroom. You may also need to assist her in basic movements until she can regain her strength. Don't shy away from helping in these ways; embrace them as a means of becoming closer. You'll also be witnessing your wife's steady progress as she becomes stronger and can once again regain her strength and independence.

Every one of these ideas will play a vital role in your wife's recovery. She may not express how much she needs you or appreciates you, but don't let that be a hindrance. Be present. Make sure she knows you are available.

And you will discover that you are doing a great work, too.

Space for a Purpose

In addition to your presence, it is equally vital that you provide the necessary space and quiet time your wife will need. Every woman will eventually want to find a quiet center where she can do her own research, meditate or pray, or simply rest. You can also help her to carve out this time.

If you have younger children at home, be sure to offer to take them to their various functions at school or help them with homework. Try to take as many events and commitments off your wife's plate as possible, and make sure she knows that her quiet time is important. There may a place in the home where she can create the quiet and serenity she needs. Allow her to have this time to strengthen her body and spirit before her surgery and/or treatment. This preparatory work will be important to her recovery later.

One woman I know, following her breast cancer diagnosis, allowed her husband to create a small English-style garden in their backyard. He laid a small walking path from the back deck, built a bench, and installed a small bubbly fountain. His wife spent many hours in her garden before and after her breast cancer treatment and considers it an important ingredient in her healing.

But a space doesn't have to be this elaborate or cost money. A porch, a deck area, an outdoor bench, or even a basement room, bedroom, or private study can all serve the same purpose. The key here is quiet, and you probably have a good idea already as to where your wife can find this space.

On occasion, some women will crave a deeper level of quiet and may also retreat more deeply into spiritual disciplines or practices. Some may feel their faith challenged or even reawakened. Toward that end, some may desire to spend more time in a church or other place of worship, while others may desire the quiet of a retreat center. Some may also want to talk to a pastor or spiritual director about the diagnosis and begin receiving the prayers of others. This in itself can be strengthening, and there have been multiple studies that show how prayer helps in the healing process.

You may also find that your wife will appreciate a writing journal, a devotional of some sort, or even some soothing music. Every woman is different. But most women will draw into a place inside where they can regain a balance and refresh their spirits. You can be of great help by providing the tools and the space she will need.

I have known many women who kept a journal of their thoughts and reflections following their breast cancer diagnosis. These were all unique. But many women find that writing their thoughts can be a form of self-analysis and introspection. Through their journals, women can discover what their hopes are and set goals that will assist them in the arduous weeks following a surgery. They may also begin to think through some of their feelings about losing a breast(s), or what their fears are, or how they believe the breast cancer will affect the way they feel about their careers, their families, or even their sexuality. A journal can be one way women can do the psychological and spiritual work of healing.

Some men may also find that journaling is helpful. Many men have the same fears women have around a breast cancer diagnosis. You may wonder:

- If my wife loses a breast, how will this affect our sexuality?

- Will I feel differently about my wife following a surgery?

- How long will it be before our lives are back to "normal"?

- Will I have the fortitude to give my wife what she needs in the days ahead?

- How will this diagnosis impact my career?

- How will the diagnosis impact our marriage? Our children?

All of these questions are legitimate, and they are questions men commonly ask. So don't overlook the need to explore your own feelings. You may also need to find a friend to talk to.

Finally, be certain to help your wife make preparations that may be needed prior to a surgery or, as you look down the longer road, for treatments and recovery. There may be items you need to purchase, a bag you need to pack. Begin talking about some of these arrangements; you might even create a list of people to call before, during and after the surgery.

As always, it doesn't hurt to have a box of some of your favorite things, too. Perhaps there are some books, candies, magazines or crossword puzzles that can help you pass the time during the procedure. Your wife may also appreciate a special recovery box filled with items that will lift her spirits. Many women, for example, treasure a photo of the family by their bedside. It never hurts to bring along the visual reminders of family and love ... especially to the hospital.

Talk about all of these things, and be sure you are creating the time and the space your wife needs as she begins her journey.

Friendship With a Purpose

Once your wife's friends learn of her cancer diagnosis, they will want to be supportive. Make sure you offer your wife plenty of time and opportunity to spend time with friends. These times will be relaxing and refreshing to her, and you can invite her friends to help in the healing process, too.

For example, some may want to cook a meal for you following your wife's surgery or during her treatments. These small gifts can mean a lot to your wife, and also to you. Having some extra food on hand can actually be a godsend, and meals will not be a worry. These friends may also wish to write letters of support or bring by other gifts. All of it can be a helpful addition to the healing process.

Likewise, invite your wife's friends to send her notes of encouragement.

Amazingly, we find that a steady dose of these positive thoughts and comments has a remarkable impact upon our mindset and our well-being. Positive thoughts really do breed positive results. And by including your wife's friends in this process as much as possible, you can be assured that she is receiving a steady dose of good words.

Although too many visits can be a bad thing, especially immediately following a surgery or during a long spell of treatments, a man can work to schedule these at appropriate intervals. There's nothing wrong with groups of people visiting when your wife is most energetic, and you will quickly learn when these times are.

Don't forget to incorporate your wife's friends into this healing mix, and do all you can to encourage her to talk about her needs. Friendship means so much through every step of the breast cancer journey.

Work With a Purpose

You can also help your wife (or mother, sister or girlfriend) by working. And work is something men know how to do. In fact, many of us work too much!

Consider, for example, the house itself—or more specifically, the housework.

Initially, when a woman learns that she has breast cancer, she will not have the same focus or energy for domestic pursuits. For a time she may feel tired, depressed or at loose ends. She won't have the same desire to tackle a load of laundry or run a cycle of dishes. In essence, she's going to need more help around the house. Even if you and your wife have always divided these chores in a kind of 50/50 proposition, you may need to carry a heavier load for a time. Where breast cancer is concerned, it's time to man up!

Since most men enjoy athletics, a sports analogy might prove helpful as an explanation. Like a football game, a man might consider how often his wife is carrying the ball when it comes to laundry, cleaning, cooking and the litany of household chores. She is likely in the game a great deal, and many of the plays are being run through her. But now she's injured. Sure, she could play tough and take one for the team and continue to carry the ball, but she would probably prefer to sit on the sidelines for a while until she can recuperate from the injury. Here's where the man can come off the bench, run with the ball for a while, take some of the pounding, and be a team player. In fact, he might even get tougher himself and learn some new skills.

Well, you get the picture. This is one of the first things a woman will need: practical help. She really won't ask for much along these lines, and some women, in fact, may actually take solace or comfort in staying busy with household chores. Laundry, cooking, cleaning ... perhaps these will be distractions for her while she is sorting out her diagnosis and prognosis in her mind. She might even become *more* busy. She might do chores she has never done before.

But here, a rule of thumb applies: be sure you are offering to help. The offer can mean as much to her as the extra hands. But if she doesn't see the willingness, it's like placing an extra burden on her back. Offer to give her the space and time she will need to rest, refresh and recharge her batteries for the real work ahead of her, which is the hard work of healing.

Men should never underestimate their role in this regard. A man can be just as much a part of the healing process as the doctors, nurses and pastors who are overseeing her physical, emotional and spiritual care. A man can provide all of these energies, too. And where love is found, there is much strength to heal.

Recently, a friend of mine posted a Facebook entry that contained some of her thoughts about her breast cancer diagnosis and subsequent surgery and recovery. She offered some bullet points of gratitude. Amazingly, in addition to thanking her surgeons and their skills, she noted that her husband was her true inspiration and source of healing. Her husband kept the household running smoothly, began cooking, and was taking the children to school every morning during her recovery period. And more than that, while she was going through her chemotherapy (and was consequently losing her hair), her husband told her every day that she was beautiful. These small acts and expressions were huge to her. And as she stated, they were, in fact, the true source of her healing.

Stay focused on the practical. Don't get sidetracked by abstract ideas or worry about what might be. Rather, dig in and lend a hand. What you do day by day will be a major source of strength and will provide your wife with amazing resiliency. Through you, she will be stronger and better able to face the challenges that are ahead of her, whatever they may be.

Helping Her Feel Good About Herself

There are a great many aspects to the breast cancer journey that can deflate your wife and make her feel somehow less of a woman, or even dejected about her marriage, her parenting or her future. All of the work you are doing will have a huge impact on lifting her.

So let's talk about a few of those pieces of the breast cancer journey that can often deflate women—and what you can do to help.

First, if your wife is going to have a mastectomy, make sure you provide plenty of opportunities for her to talk about what the loss of the breast means. Not just for her, but for you, too. You can help her to realize that the loss of the breast is not the end of your marriage or your sexual chemistry. The best is yet to come!

If a breast cancer diagnosis is part of a larger history in her family—maybe her mother died of cancer—work hard to reassure her that medicine continues to advance and change. The past does not dictate the future. Likewise, do your best to provide reminders that there is a life ahead (family photos, important dates on your calendar, anniversaries, vacations, trips you are planning). Give her these goals to strive for, and reassure her that you are looking forward to sharing these times with her. You expect her to be there. The cancer is not a death sentence.

Some women may also fear lymphedema (a painful swelling of the arm following lymph node treatment). Lymphedema, of course, does not affect all women; even among those who have lymph node radiation or chemotherapy, it does not always occur. Remind her of the information her physicians have given her, and direct her to some of the lymphedema support Web sites that can answer her questions or set her mind at ease.

One of the most troublesome aspects of chemotherapy is hair loss. This side effect of the healing process can often make a woman shy away from interaction with others or even embarrass her. If your wife must take a type of chemotherapy that may result in hair loss, however, you can be her cheerleader and confidant. There are several things you can do that can actually make her feel better about herself.

First, many women are surprised at how pervasive the support becomes when she loses her hair. Her children may want to shave their heads (would you?) in order to demonstrate solidarity. Sometimes a woman's friends will follow suit, too. And before you know it, you've got many people in your corner sporting the swimmer's look. Remind your wife that her hair loss is just a part of the healing process and that, as she completes her therapy and her hair begins to grow back, it will be a reminder of how far she has come and how quickly the healing is progressing.

You can also help your wife through this hair-loss period by supplying her with some new hats, scarves, do-rags and even wigs. Your oncologist can recommend some to you; there are even clothiers and suppliers who are dedicated to women's chemotherapy fashion. Search the web and you'll find more than you bargained for!

Finally, a woman who is going through hair loss will benefit from soothing lotions and oils. Again, check with your oncologist regarding the best options here, but you will be able to find some wonderful bath oils and scented candles that can give your wife a sensory experience and make her feel refreshed and energized. These small gifts can keep her spirit strong and help her realize how much you care.

If you want to go beyond the lotions and oils, make your wife a coupon book and offer to massage her back, shoulders, neck and arms when she needs the soothing comfort of your touch. You could also find a massage therapist in your area; there are some who actually specialize in post-cancer massage for women.

All of these can be tremendous gifts that can lift your wife's spirit and set her on a fast road to recovery.

Become a Nutrition and Exercise Guru

Men can help their wives by becoming more aware of their nutritional and physical requirements. Again, this doesn't have to be anything extraordinary, just helpful. But when a woman receives a breast cancer diagnosis, she will need to begin thinking about her nutritional and physical goals. Every situation, every diagnosis, every prognosis is different. However, every physician will eventually create a plan, whether it is surgery, radiation, chemotherapy or some combination, and nutrition and strength will be a part of that preparation and recovery process.

Your physician can guide you further in these needs—and make recommendations—but women will do well to take a multivitamin and drink plenty of water in this preparation time.

Again, a doctor is your true source of information here, and don't forget to ask about nutrition. The doctor may even prescribe a pre-surgery, pre-treatment diet. But don't overlook the role you can play in creating some healthy meals to help her stay focused on her health goals. Eat what she eats, especially if the diet is new to you.

One woman I know—a breast cancer survivor of twelve years—became a vegetarian during her surgery prep period. And during her recovery phase she began hiking as a means of recovering her strength. She has continued these pursuits—this lifestyle—long into her cancer-free years, but she attributes her new life to these disciplines.

This is not to say that you and your wife must become vegetarians or take up hiking. Far from it. The point is simply that every man can help his wife maintain the focus and discipline necessary to eat and sleep her way toward health.

Exercise (especially stretching) is important, too.

If surgery is involved in the healing, then some of these prescribed exercises and stretches could be incorporated into a routine beforehand. Performing these movements before the surgery will only enhance and hasten the recovery afterward. Again, your doctor will know what these exercises will be, so inquire. And then help your wife become familiar with them.

If your wife is already an exercise buff, encourage her to continue these exercises as long as possible before her treatment. These movements and disciplines will keep her strong and help her relieve stress, too. She will be able to work out her tensions on the treadmill. Give her the space and the time to pursue these workouts so she can stay strong ... and you stay strong with her.

Don't be surprised if your wife enjoys sex with more frequency, too. It is often the case that tensions and stresses—particularly medical issues—can make couples retreat into intimacy more often. She may, in fact, find sex to be another one of these stress relievers. Don't overlook sexual intimacy as another way to be present and supportive—in fact, your wife may actually crave your touch, your physical warmth. She may take solace in a deeper intimacy. And you won't want to disappoint. Many couples discover that their sexual energy and intensity is heightened after breast cancer (is this a survivalist instinct?). So don't be surprised if your wife discovers a newfound passion.

There are many ways you can help your wife become more aware of her progress, too. Always encourage her verbally, and if she needs help with her exercises or needs motivation, don't hesitate to do the movements with her. Eat what she eats. Stay positive.

Day by day you will see progress in both the preparatory phase and afterward. You can also make a chart to help you stay focused on the goals, and it never hurts to create a daily menu if you have certain nutritional instructions. If medication is required, make a chart or create a refrigerator calendar that can help your wife stay on track with her various prescriptions. Do whatever is needed to assist your wife in her progress, and point out how well she is doing.

Summary

Every man can learn how to be present and supportive during his wife's illness. He doesn't have to fix the problem; he just has to be accounted for.

Small efforts can add up to big gifts when a woman is going through breast cancer. She will note these, and in her heart she will be grateful.

ॐ

First Person

I'm not sure what advice I would give for others going through this, but I do think most men don't want to talk about the breast cancer experience. They certainly don't seem very eager to talk to other men about it.

But I think that would be a very helpful thing, actually ... to talk to other men and compare notes. Well, not compare notes, perhaps, but certainly to commiserate. I think talking about these things helps immensely. It's a way to help ourselves, not just our wives.

I guess I would recommend that men talk to their friends. In fact, this will make them better friends.

If there was anything I did try to do for my wife, it was this: I tried to stay positive along the way. I think my wife, like many women, often lived in a dark cloud during that time—especially during the long months of therapy—and so I always tried to help her see the bright side of the healing process. I had to work at it, actually—I'm not naturally a positive person—but I kept my fears to myself, and I never did share these with my wife. So, I was changed, too. And the positive attitude definitely impacted me.

I don't recall doing a lot of things differently around the house. I think my wife still wanted to do some of the chores; perhaps it was her own therapy, although I did do extra work from time to time when she was too tired. But primarily we tried to keep as much of our daily routines as possible. Consistency was important.

A lot of people seem to blame God when they receive a breast cancer diagnosis, but I never did go there. I saw God as helper, as support. I think this was crucial to our outlook and positive healing, too.

I think the main thing I'd recommend for other men in this situation is that they find someone to talk to. It might be difficult, but it can be very important for their own peace of mind.

~Bob

Five Things to Remember

- Your presence is far more important than trying to fix the problem. Be present with your wife and attend all of the appointments with her.

- Give her space.

- Allow friends to help.

- Take on more responsibilities around the house.

- Become a nutrition and exercise junkie.

Ten Gifts You Can Give

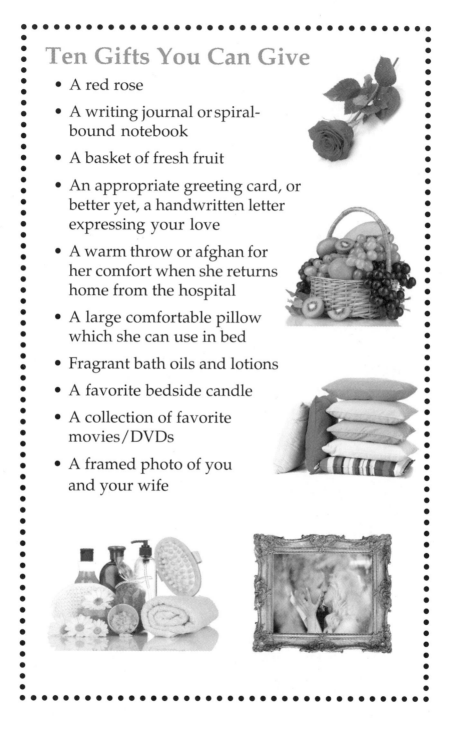

- A red rose

- A writing journal or spiral-bound notebook

- A basket of fresh fruit

- An appropriate greeting card, or better yet, a handwritten letter expressing your love

- A warm throw or afghan for her comfort when she returns home from the hospital

- A large comfortable pillow which she can use in bed

- Fragrant bath oils and lotions

- A favorite bedside candle

- A collection of favorite movies/DVDs

- A framed photo of you and your wife

Chapter Three
What is Breast Cancer?

Breast cancer is a very complex disease, and because it is also unique to the individual, diagnosis, prognosis, treatment(s) and even descriptions can vary from person to person. And as medicine, knowledge and treatments continue to adapt, even the language and terminology that doctors use to describe breast cancer can vary by individual.

In essence, however, breast cancer begins when normal cells in the breast change to an uncontrolled growth pattern. This abnormal growth usually begins in the smallest form—sometimes only in the milk ducts—but can spread to other parts of the breast or even to other tissues and organs such as the lymph nodes or beyond. When these cancer cells grow and expand to distant sites in the body, the process is called **metastasis**.

Doctors will generally describe breast cancer as a **carcinoma**, but there are, in fact, many types of breast cancers, appearing in different parts of the breast. Not all of these cancers develop into **tumors**, which could generally be described as cancerous growths. Moreover, not all breast cancers grow at the same rate. Some forms are aggressive, meaning they grow rapidly. Other forms develop very slowly. And again, each cancer will grow and develop at varying rates depending upon the individual, the individual's age, overall health, and many other factors.

One thing that men need to keep in mind, however, is that a breast cancer diagnosis is usually not a medical emergency. In most cases, a woman has time to consider her options for treatment and to select a surgeon and hospital, and can weigh many other factors before committing to a surgery or treatment. Second opinions may be sought.

A man can help through this entire process, too, especially by being levelheaded and affirming. After the initial diagnosis, a man can be most helpful by taking a step back, staying positive, and doing his own research.

One man describes his own reaction to his wife's breast cancer diagnosis this way:

"My initial reaction was shock. I thought a breast cancer diagnosis was a death sentence. But as the doctor explained the realities and the treatment options, I realized that my wife's prognosis was very good, that she would be able to have a surgery and live a normal life. Once I understood what breast cancer was—or in my wife's case, what is wasn't—I really dug in and began thinking of all the things she would need, all the things I could do for her, and this really helped me, too. It gave me a job to do. And the more I read about breast cancer, the more I understood what my wife was going through and what she would need from me. Ask questions. Always ask questions."

Understanding breast cancer is important. And while there are many types of breast cancers, it might be helpful to describe some of the basic forms. See the diagram on the facing page for a brief explanation of the four most common forms.

Again, a breast cancer diagnosis is rarely a medical emergency. Most likely the first suggestion of breast cancer will be detection from a mammogram. Usually this is followed by a biopsy, and thereafter a doctor will use this information (along with the mammogram or other image testing) to determine the type of cancer and treatment options.

In some cases, surgery will be the only treatment needed. In other cases, surgery will be followed by subsequent treatments of radiation, chemotherapy, or hormonal therapy. The biopsy report and the doctor's expertise will be determining factors in the pathology report, and together the doctor and patient will plot a course for healing.

Sometimes doctors will describe breast cancer as localized (in the breast only), regional (having spread to the nodes near the breast), or distant (having spread to other organs or regions of the body). Sometimes these various cancers are described as stages, with Stage 1 being the most localized or confined and Stage 4 being the most serious, or having spread to other parts of the body.

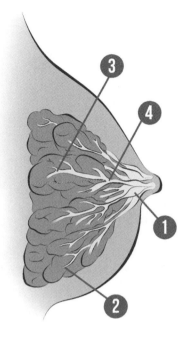

Ductal carcinomas (#1) begin in the milk ducts of the breast, and in very early forms, may remain **in situ,** meaning the cancer is contained inside the walls of the duct (or lobular) and has not invaded the surrounding tissue. Ductal carcinomas are the most common, and when detected early, are highly treatable.

Lobular carcinomas (#2) begin in the breast lobules (where milk is produced) and are less common than ductal cancers.

Infiltrating lobular carcinoma (#3) means the cancer has infiltrated the breast tissue outside the lobular gland.

Infiltrating ductal carcinoma (#4) means the cancer has infiltrated the breast tissue outside the milk duct.

The more you and your wife understand about the cancer, the better informed you will be to make decisions regarding treatment and recovery time. As was mentioned earlier in the testimony, ask lots of questions. Always ask the doctor to explain something further if you don't understand.

Understanding the Specifics

Because there are many questions you could (and probably *should*) ask your surgeon, it may be helpful to include here some of the most common—especially if you have yet to discuss treatment options openly and are reading this book prior to a first visit with the surgeon or care team. These questions are important ones and can serve as a springboard to some questions of your own that you'd like your physician to answer.

- What type of breast cancer is this?

- If there is a tumor, what size is it?

- Is the cancer contained (in situ) or has is spread outside the duct/lobular walls (invasive)?

- Has the cancer spread to the lymph nodes, and is there a way to determine this for certain?

- Is the cancer only in one area of the breast, or multiple?

- Is there cancer in the other breast?

- What can you tell us about this type of cancer and odds of survivability?

- Could the cancer return after treatment?

- How aggressive is this cancer or tumor? (How fast does it generally grow?)

- What else can you tell us about this cancer that we should know?

Initially, when a woman receives the diagnosis of her breast cancer, she may experience fear, isolation, frustration, confusion, guilt, anxiety or even denial. These reactions are understandable, and every woman is different in her approach as she works through these feelings.

Understanding breast cancer is one of the most helpful aspects of the healing process, and without solid information, it is far more difficult for women to make subsequent choices regarding their treatment and reconstructive surgery (if this is an option). A man can help by listening closely to what the doctor is saying, taking notes, and even providing information to his wife that may help her in this process of discernment.

Likewise, a man will also have his own emotional baggage to contend with. A breast cancer diagnosis may make him feel powerless, fearful or angry. And if there are marital stresses, the diagnosis may bring these to the forefront of the relationship. A man will need to be aware of these feelings but also find a way to assist in the conversations and the healing process.

So, when we ponder the question, *What is breast cancer?*, we also see that the disease is not only physical but also relational. We can describe the disease in medical detail, but there are deeper ramifications, too.

Some years ago, soon after my cousin's breast cancer diagnosis (and her subsequent death due to metastatic cancer), I recall talking to her husband about this experience. He told me:

"No marriage is perfect, but I felt that this breast cancer was also impacting me. When I learned how serious this cancer was, I was afraid. We had to find new ways to talk about the disease and our future. As the disease progressed, I felt very lonely."

Don't forget: the two of you are going through this together. Understanding the medical procedures is only a part of the equation. Understanding each other is just as crucial.

Additional Facts

Once your wife begins to discuss the surgical procedure with the doctor, it will be helpful to have visuals at hand. No doubt the doctor can and will provide this through brochures, videos or even medical books.

In addition, you may hear terms like "stage" or "tumor size" and wonder what these mean. To give you a basic understanding, I have included a quick reference guide to tumor size and the stages of cancer that doctors often use. **Please consult your doctor, however, about all of these points**! Every breast cancer case is different in form and complexity, so make certain you understand each point your physician is relaying.

Tumors

Remember that not all breast cancers are in tumor form, but if your doctor is talking about a tumor, the following may give you some perspective.

.43 to 1.1 centimeters	Tumor is the size of a pea
.59 to 1.5 centimeters	Tumor is the size of a dime
.81 to 2.1 centimeters	Tumor is the size of a nickel
1.4 to 3.6 centimeters	Tumor is the size of a quarter

Stages

Medical nomenclature and knowledge continue to adapt and morph, but in the event your doctor is discussing a "stage" of cancer, here is a quick guide. Again, your doctor is the expert on these stages and can tell you much more, so use this guide only as a point of conversation with the physician.

Stage 0

This means noninvasive breast cancer (in situ). The abnormal or pre-cancerous cells are inside a globule or milk duct, but there is no evidence the cancer has "broken free" of the duct and invaded surrounding tissue.

Stage 1

This is the first stage of "invasive" breast cancer, which means the cancer cells have invaded surrounding tissue within the breast. The tumor(s) is of a small size and in the breast(s) only. No lymph nodes are involved.

Stage 2

This stage means that the tumor(s) is between 2 and 5 centimeters and may or may not have spread to the lymph nodes.

Physicians will generally tell the patient about the size and location of this tumor as detected.

Stage 3

This stage means that the tumor is 5 centimeters or larger and may have spread to the lymph nodes, the chest wall, or to other places surrounding the breast. Again, a doctor can generally parse this stage and clarify the invasiveness and location of the tumor. Ask.

Stage 4

This stage involves a tumor of any size that has spread beyond the breast region and has invaded other areas of the body (lungs, liver, bone, brain, etc.). Often this stage is referred to as "metastatic."

Understanding the Surgery Options

Mastectomy Procedures

The illustration below can help you understand the various forms of lumpectomies and mastectomies. Be sure to clarify these terms and procedures with your surgeon. In the next chapter, you will find additional questions that can assist you in your discussion about these important matters. If the surgeon does not provide you with brochures, you can use some of these illustrations to get you started. The surgeon can clarify any of these procedures and what the pros and cons are for each of them.

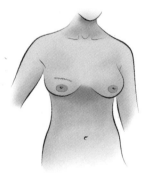

Lumpectomy surgery with scar

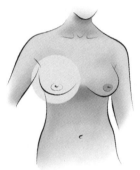

Mastectomy (area to be surgically removed in highlight)

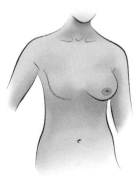

Post-mastectomy (with scar)

Understanding the Lumpectomy

The lumpectomy has often been described as a breast-conserving surgery. It differs from the mastectomy in the amount of tissue removed, but it is not an option for all women. A lumpectomy *may be* an option, but only if your doctor recommends it. Be sure to ask your surgeon about the reasons why a lumpectomy may or may not be an option for your wife.

To help in your discussion, here is a basic description of the lumpectomy surgery.

A lumpectomy removes the tumor and a small wedge of surrounding tissue. In some procedures, a second wedge of tissue may be removed from under the arm(s) where the lymph nodes are found.

Commonly, a lumpectomy will *not* be recommended if any of the following conditions apply:

- Other calcifications or tumors are revealed in other parts of the breast or in more than one location.

- The type of cancer suggests a more aggressive surgery.

- The size of the tumor is such that larger margins would be required to increase the likelihood of cure and recovery.

- The location of the calcifications or tumor suggests a more aggressive surgery.

- The tumor is in proximity to the lymph nodes.

- There is a greater possibility that the calcifications have spread, or could spread, to other regions of the breast.

- There has been prior radiation to the breast or the breast area.

- The woman has had a chronic lung disease.

- There is a genetic predisposition to breast cancer or a family history of breast cancer.

Naturally, many women will want to know if a lumpectomy (versus a mastectomy) is an option. Many women will want to know if their breasts can be preserved, at least in part. So when you go with your wife to see the surgeon, this is likely to be one of the questions she will ask.

I recall that, during our conversation with the surgeon, the lumpectomy option was indeed batted around for a time. I also recall the surgeon handing us a pamphlet that contained the pros and cons of lumpectomies and mastectomies, and much of our initial conversation centered on asking questions about the options available.

Some of these pros and cons follow:

Lumpectomy PROS

- A lumpectomy can preserve body image by saving a larger portion of the breast, which could include the nipple and areola.

- The woman can continue to wear her own bra.

- The hospitalization and recovery time is less.

- A lumpectomy may be easier to accept psychologically and emotionally.

- A lumpectomy can be effective in some situations, and it does not affect survival rate in those situations where a lumpectomy is appropriate, although a second surgery (a mastectomy) may be required in the future if the cancer does return. This can prove traumatic and should be considered in the decision to have a lumpectomy.

Lumpectomy CONS

- There is always a risk of recurrence in the remaining breast tissue.

- When a woman ops for a lumpectomy, she will usually couple this with some radiation treatments of the surrounding breast tissue.

- After radiation therapy, there can be a noticeable difference in feel and appearance of the breast.

- The breast where the lumpectomy was performed will have a noticeable difference in appearance from the other breast (size, shape, texture, etc.).

- The monthly self-exam of the lumpectomy breast will be more difficult because of the radiation therapy.

- If the lumpectomy and radiation are not effective, a second surgery and treatment may be required.

Mastectomy PROS

- The mastectomy removes most of the breast tissue (including nipple and areola) and thus reduces a cancer recurrence significantly.

- Reconstruction of the breast is possible using the woman's own tissues from elsewhere in the body or by breast implant(s).

- A breast implant (along with nipple reconstruction and tattooing) can restore the mastectomy breast to a similar size and shape to the remaining, thus making it possible for the woman to wear her own bras.

Mastectomy CONS

- A woman's body image is altered because of the surgery.

- There will be a need for a prosthesis or reconstruction with tissue or implant.

- The recovery time for a mastectomy is generally longer than with a lumpectomy, and subsequent visits to the plastic surgeon for reconstruction (tattooing) may be required.

- A mastectomy does not guarantee that there will not be a recurrence of cancer.

Hopefully this comparison can provide some preliminary information for you and your wife to ponder as you continue your discussion and review with the surgeon. No decision should be made in isolation. Be aware that your wife will have much stronger feelings about these options than you do. One of these choices will impact her more deeply. You can help her consider what the surgeon has detailed and remind her of what options are or are not available to her. Clarity will be important.

Reconstruction Options

In the event that your wife selects a reconstructive option, she will want to weigh her choice carefully. Naturally, every plastic surgeon has a preference and can help your wife make an informed decision. Most women do opt for some form of reconstructive work, which can certainly assist in the recovery process.

As far as reconstruction is concerned, again there are options, both in terms of timing and technique. Some women prefer to have, for example, a mastectomy and the initial stages of reconstruction (whether tissue transfer or implant) accomplished during the one surgery. In this timing, the pathologist surgeon and plastic surgeon work as a team, with the mastectomy and subsequent repairs being made under the same anesthesia. In fact, many surgeons work out of the same medical group or in conjunction with each other in this fashion. Usually your breast surgeon can recommend a plastic surgeon and may even have a partner who completes this second stage of the surgery.

Other women may opt to have the reconstructive phase completed later—even after several weeks. She may feel this timing is better for her or will give her a greater ability to adapt to the changes in her body.

As for techniques or reconstructive methods, there are several options of tissue transfer. One involves the transfer of stomach muscle (*rectus abdominus*). Here a portion of abdominal muscle is removed from the woman's body and transplanted into the breast area. The goal is to form a breast of size and shape similar to the other. In this procedure, there will be scarring, of course, in both the breast area and in the abdomen. Women who undergo this procedure will generally have moderate pain for several weeks in the abdominal and chest areas.

Another option involves removing a portion of back muscle (*latissimus dorsi* or lat) and transplanting it to the breast. The technique is much the same as the one used for the stomach muscle transplant. Following the back muscle transplant, the woman will have pain in the chest and back for weeks following this surgery.

A third option, though far less used, involves removing tissue from other places in the body such as the buttocks or thighs.

In any of these procedures, when a mastectomy has first been performed, the plastic surgeon will reconstruct a nipple and areola from the woman's own tissues. The skin is molded to the shape and size of the other nipple and is grafted into the reconstructed breast. (Tattooing usually comes later and involves making the reconstructed nipple the same hue as the other.)

As you and your wife consider these options for reconstruction, there are many considerations to weigh. No doubt she will grow to have a strong affinity for one over the other, and you can assist her in supporting this decision.

Here is a quick guide that can assist you in weighing the options and the timing of the reconstruction. Be sure to review this with your plastic surgeon as well, as he/she will likely have a specialty and an opinion about which will work best for your wife's situation. You can find questions for the plastic surgeon in the next chapter, and these can serve as a guide for your conversation about these matters.

Breast Implant PROS

- Breast implants have been around for many years now and are used by millions of women.

- A breast implant can be expanded to closely resemble the size and shape—and even texture—of the other breast.

- Breast implants do provide options for women in terms of increased (or decreased) size.

- Implants can be removed.

- Implants do not require invasive surgeries to other parts of the body (such as the abdomen, back or buttocks).

- Recovery time is reduced because an invasive surgery to the abdomen or back is not being performed.

- The cost is usually lower because only one surgery is necessary, in contrast to a second surgery needed to remove tissues.

Breast Implant CONS

- Every implant will eventually need to be replaced (though some implants do have a longer cycle than expected).

- Breast implants can be punctured (due to a heavy blow to the chest or an injury).

- Breast implants are not "fool proof" (there are slight risks).

- Because they are not tissue, breast implants may feel foreign to some women.

As far as timing for reconstruction, here is a quick guide for your discussion with the surgeon. No doubt he/she can give you much more information, but will likely share similar thoughts.

Reconstruction at the Time of Mastectomy PROS

- Only one surgery and anesthesia is needed.

- The woman will not have to "gear herself up" for two surgeries.

- Immediately after the mastectomy the woman will have a "new" breast, not later.

- The recovery time is reduced.

- The full recovery period is reduced (no waiting for a second surgery).

- There is less risk involved in one surgery vs. two, and less cost.

Reconstruction at the Time of Mastectomy CONS

- There is more initial physical discomfort and more impact to the body at one time.

- The initial surgery is longer.

- There is slightly more risk that there will be complications due to the reconstructive phase.

Reconstruction Delayed PROS

- Women who feel "hurried" can have more time to consider their options following a mastectomy.

- There is no potential delay in treatments (radiation or chemotherapy).

- A woman will have time to study the reconstructive options available to her and won't be making any decision based on fear or insistence of others.

- Some women may decide not to have reconstruction at all, but opt for a prosthesis instead.

Reconstruction Delayed CONS

- A second surgery is required.

- There is agreater cost due to a second surgery and all the accompanying amenities (anesthesia, operating room, hospital room, nursing, etc.).

- Having no reconstruction for some weeks or having to wear a temporary prosthesis may feel like an inconvenience to some women. Some insurance plans may not cover a second surgery on delay, or a second deductible may have to be met. Careful review of your insurance plan and consultation with a representative is recommended.

- There may be additional costs between the first surgery and second surgery (special bras, two sets of drainage tubes, etc.).

- There is a greater potential for fear or worry because a second surgery is required.

- Self-image may be impacted by waiting, and a woman can't hasten the process once the mastectomy has been performed.

Preparing for Surgery

Once your wife has made a decision about surgery and/or reconstruction, she will have a surgery date set and will eventually have a pre-admission assessment. This assessment is usually closer to the surgery time and will include blood work, a complete health history and a review of all the surgery procedures. Knowing about these surgery procedures—including the length of the operation and the protocol the doctors will follow—will be important for your peace of mind, too.

I recall that, before my wife's surgery, I drove to the hospital to make certain I knew where to park and where the waiting room and cafeteria were located. I was also shown a small waiting room where the surgeon would meet with me in private immediately following the surgery to give me an update on the mastectomy and the implant. This "walk-through" gave me peace of mind and actually helped me immensely on the day of the surgery, as I did not have to ask questions or wander about the hospital in search of a cup of coffee or a magazine rack. I also had a general idea about the location of my wife's room following the surgery and was able to make some minor preparations in the room before her arrival. I had also arranged a cot in my wife's room so I could spend the night, and I was able to inform all of our family and friends about the outcome before my wife arrived in her room.

I would recommend this type of walk-through.

Men would also do well to make a list of pre-surgery items their wives will need. (She will likely have this list, too, provided by the hospital.) Men can also create their own overnight bags that could include items like reading materials, reading glasses, a cell phone charger, toiletries, cash for the cafeteria, and contact numbers for family and friends. Collecting all of these materials (and other personal items) before the day of the surgery will also give you more time to focus on your wife's needs. She may need to talk or perhaps sit quietly in the hours leading up to the surgery. Being prepared will save you a great deal of scurrying about later.

If your wife's surgery requires an overnight stay (a mastectomy), you will want to be aware of several other realities.

The day of the surgery may be difficult for your wife, so plan to make her as comfortable as possible. She will not have eaten for many hours and will no doubt be hungry and thirsty, so I would recommend you save your own appetite for the hours of the surgery itself, when you can take a break with some coffee or a snack and await word from the surgeon. You will probably not feel like eating, anyway, and there's a certain affinity that husbands share with their wives during these times.

When your wife returns to her room after surgery, she will still be groggy from the anesthesia. Allow her to remain quiet and still as much as possible, buffer visitors as needed, and remain by her side while she comes out of the anesthesia.

Many women, in the hours following, may feel not only groggy, but also nauseous. Although she may be offered food, she may not feel like eating. Some women do well with anesthesia, while others do not. If your wife is nauseous or is vomiting, you may need to assist her with cleanup, as she will not be able to move her arm(s). She will be relatively immobile for a few hours.

Post Hospital Prep

Before you leave the hospital, the nurse will likely remove the bandaging and show you and your wife how to change the dressing and administer the drainage tube. This can be a very traumatic time for your wife, when she glimpses the scar for the first time. Although she may have seen many photographs of other scars or read about the surgery in the various brochures, seeing her own body can be difficult. And if your wife has had a mastectomy followed by reconstruction under the same anesthesia, she may not yet have a nipple on the breast. Again, she should be prepared for this, but it can nevertheless be shocking.

The nurse may give you instructions, as the caregiver, on how to change the dressing on the breast and how to help your wife with a shower. You may have already reviewed these matters with the surgeon, but watch and listen carefully as the nurse walks through the process with you. And again, make sure you have enough gauze and wrappings at home. This will be a valuable part of your prep work. Your wife's room at home should also be prepared and stocked.

Take some time before the day of surgery to make your car ready for your wife's transfer from the hospital (usually via wheelchair). Don't wait until the last minute to clean debris from the seat or the floorboard; have her seat area cleaned and ready to go before you get to the car. Make sure the seatbelt works easily and properly. Drive carefully.

Once at home, you should be able to transfer your wife from the car to her room without having to worry about clutter on the floor or on the steps. Another family member might want to assist you. Make sure her steps are safe and sure as you get her to bed.

In many ways this last step—seeing your wife back home—is a great relief. You will feel that you have overcome the first (and perhaps last) of the hurdles. There truly is no place like home, and your wife will be able to begin her healing journey in the comfort of her own bed, surrounded by love and attention. She will be able to rest more soundly, and you will see, day by day, that your wife is making progress and getting stronger.

Make certain you follow the doctor's orders and any schedule of medication your wife needs, and give her a helping hand—at least for the first few days—with showering, going to the bathroom, and making her way around the house. Initially, assist her in her exercises, as well.

The journey is just beginning, but in many ways you have already crossed the most important threshold. Stay positive and focused, and your wife will respond in kind.

From Understanding to Decision

As most doctors will point out, the majority of breast cancer cases do not require a series of immediate decisions (as in hours or a few days). In most instances, a woman will have time to weigh her options, process information, and even gather other opinions if she desires. She can talk to other breast cancer survivors. She can reflect and center herself to make a wise and informed choice.

Sometimes a woman needs more than one conversation with a doctor. Early on, when a woman is still in a state of shock or disbelief, she may miss bits and pieces of information the doctor is sharing. Her fear may get the best of her. You can help, of course, by taking notes during these visits and attempting to ply certain bullet points and key concepts onto paper for her. There may be books or pamphlets the doctor recommends for reading. There may be a DVD to watch.

Many doctors will prefer a follow-up visit to review the procedures and make certain the patient understands all of the risks and implications of any choice. The doctor may, in fact, have a recommendation, and many women are looking for a doctor to give them this direction. Don't feel that you have to remain silent on the matter or interject your opinion quickly. Be sure to let your wife process the information on her own. Allow her to bounce questions off you. Help her with her research. Help her to understand breast cancer as best you can.

Don't forget to remind your wife that she can always call the doctor if she has follow-up questions. Most doctors will be available in this way or will provide an Internet option or a Web site for such questions at the end of each day. Some doctors may even provide a cell number or may be willing to give a call back if a woman leaves a voice mail message at the office.

Finally, if your wife is having difficulty making a decision about her surgery, reconstruction options, and follow-up therapies, create a pro/con list. Weigh all of these options together, with your wife having the final say. Creating this side-by-side list of options will provide a visible and detailed procedure for making these decisions.

When my wife was weighing her options, creating this pro/con list was most valuable. In fact, we spent at least two days studying this list, praying for wisdom, and discussing the options in great detail. Nothing we did was more helpful in making the decision.

ഇൗരു

First Person

I was with my wife in the doctor's office when we received the news. My first reaction was fear. I suppose this was really a fear of the unknown: what this meant for us and what my wife would be facing.

Upon our return visits with the doctor—when we received a fuller diagnosis and treatment options—our daughter-in-law was there to take notes. She listed and recorded everything the doctor was saying so we could have this information for later. There was so much to absorb, so much information. Having someone else to take notes was very helpful.

In the weeks ahead—while my wife was preparing for her surgery and subsequent treatments (radiation and chemo)—I tried to be optimistic and supportive. I made it a point to reassure my wife that everything would be all right. I saw my role as providing help, being the helper. I did this in a lot of ways.

For example, during my wife's chemo sessions—there were twelve in all—she would become very dehydrated at times, and I made it a point to remind her to drink lots of water. But she also became weak, and once she had to have a blood transfusion. So it was important that I go along for all the treatments.

We were very pleased with the professional help my wife received. We had the same woman in the treatment center who helped with the chemo, and she had a wonderful sense of humor that put us at ease. She was always upbeat.

The chemo was the most difficult part. My wife actually did very well with the surgery, but the chemo is a much longer process. It felt like a long ride. Especially for her. Losing her hair was a very traumatic time for her. Women may be more self-conscious than men and may also feel that they have been disfigured. But I don't think a mastectomy changes the way a man sees his wife.

During all of these treatments, we prayed a lot—each in our own way—and our spiritual life was more intense during this time.

Following this breast cancer experience, we both have a much deeper appreciation for each day. We don't take life for granted. I think we are both more attentive and thankful for each day.

~Larry

5 Things to Remember:

- Allow your wife the necessary time and energy to make an informed decision about her surgery options.

- Be sure you understand the prognosis for your wife's "stage" of cancer.

- Consider the pros and cons of a lumpectomy versus a mastectomy.

- Consider the pros and cons of breast implants versus reconstruction.

- Make certain your wife understands the healing process and all follow-up therapies.

Husband's Quick Guide to Breast Cancer Chemo

Top 10 Things to Remember

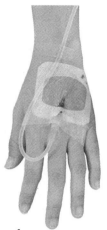

1. Not all chemotherapy is the same, and your wife may respond much differently to her treatment than do other women taking the same or different treatments.

2. Chemo has seasons to it (times of energy and times when she will feel tired or depressed).

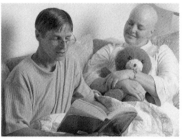

3. When possible, go with your wife to her chemotherapy treatments. This will bring you closer, and she will appreciate this extra support.

4. If your wife is going to lose her hair, consider head coverings, wigs, and hats in advance.

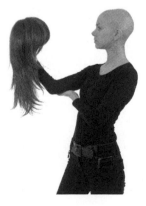

5. Consider also other signs of solidarity that you and the family could implement to help your wife when she loses her hair.

6. Remember: your wife may lose her appetite.

7. Remember: your wife may not feel sexy or in the mood during chemo.

8. Stay positive and encouraging during her treatments.

9. Chemo can seem like a long haul, so don't become impatient or removed.

10. Do something nice for your wife every week during her therapy.

Chapter Four
Your Allies in Breast Cancer

Looking back on the weeks following my wife's breast cancer diagnosis, I realize those days were the most intense and time consuming we experienced. We read a stack of books. We printed information we gleaned from the Internet. We made phone calls to arrange appointments with oncologists and surgeons. We called our insurance representative and fielded dozens of inquiries from family and friends. It was a dizzying adventure, both harrowing and exhausting. But with each decision we made, we felt a sense of peace and relaxation. Burdens lifted. A calm eventually ensued.

Most men will confirm that this initial decision-making phase of a breast cancer diagnosis is the most difficult time for them. It is also the time when men can feel the most helpful and when a steady, solid approach is most needed.

But there are decisions to be made. And lots of them.

When my wife and I began this decision-making process, we actually made some mistakes. And as they say, hindsight is 20-20. That's one of the reasons I wanted to write this book—to help men (and women) have a clearer path to making the best decisions. And there are a few insights here that I think can offer.

First, there certainly is a lot of information that can be gleaned from articles, books and even the pamphlets the physician provides. Sure, read them. Read them all. But my wife also learned a great deal from talking to other women who were recent breast cancer survivors. In fact, she readily admits that she wishes she had spent more time talking to other women about their experiences and choices. It wasn't just the support she felt, but also the information she was able to obtain from these other women, that helped immensely.

So be certain you suggest to your wife (or mother, girlfriend, sister, etc.) that she talk to other women who are in her age group, of her generation. Some of the women my wife talked to initially were much older, and while their insights were helpful, they were often not aware of the most recent developments in surgical procedures and therapies. Breast cancer treatments continue to change and adapt, so be sure that your wife is finding women who have had recent experiences. She will have no trouble finding these women if she makes a few phone calls. Breast cancer survivors are everywhere!

Second, don't assume you can make a decision about a surgeon or hospital from just one phone call, visit or a first impression. No matter where you live, there will be options for you. And if you do a bit of research and listen to the grapevine, you can ascertain what the top options are. There will be doctors who will come highly recommended. Others may have an unfavorable reputation. Same with hospitals and clinics.

Initially my wife had made a decision for her surgery (and surgeon) based on her own research and office visit. But she continued to hear from other women who suggested she talk with yet another surgeon, a doctor who was both renowned and cutting-edge in his approach to breast cancer. This surgeon, we would also learn, had a sharp wit and a sense of humor, both attributes my wife and I found refreshing.

After my wife and I visited this surgeon together one afternoon, our reactions were both the same: he was the one. His approach, demeanor and expertise were a perfect fit. My wife did an about-face, canceled her previous surgery date, phoned the other surgeon and hospital, and thanked them. Then she signed up with the other surgeon. She was glad she did.

Likewise, your wife will eventually arrive at these decisions in her own time and way. But you can help. Keep her talking. Keep her moving. And keep her thinking about her options.

Because you are not the one who has breast cancer, your work can be one of suggestion and approval. You can help her through this process of decision making by pointing out the progress she is making and helping her through the sticking points. You can help her avoid feeling overwhelmed by the number of decisions she must make.

So, let's take a quick tour of these decisions and break them down one step at a time.

The Breast Surgeon

In many respects, the breast surgeon a woman selects will be her most important choice. She will want to feel comfortable with, and confident in, this surgeon, both for his/her expertise and personality. The breast surgeon will be responsible for removing the cancerous tissue, performing this procedure well, and perhaps also removing some or even all of the breast(s). And so, the breast surgeon looms large in the frame.

The surgeon will, in many respects, be like the general in the small army of medical personnel who will be attending to your wife's needs and her future health. So your wife will want to feel confident that he/she is able to lead the team and is up to date on the latest advancements and procedures. Skill is a factor, of course. But experience and history will also play a large role in her level of comfort.

Depending upon your wife's prognosis and needs, the breast surgeon will, in many respects, be working alongside the pathologist, oncologist, radiologist and anesthesiologist. The surgeon may also have recommendations in all of these arenas, so a comfort with the surgeon can lead to other relationships in the medical community. These other specialists may also have worked closely with the surgeon in the past, so your wife may also be assembling a team of players who have worked together before. She should hope so.

As noted earlier, your wife will want to listen to the experiences of other women, and from these she will begin to hear certain names repeated. Women feel very strongly about their surgeons and their breast cancer experiences, and if a woman thinks her surgeon is tops, well, then he is ... to her. No doubt there will be many highly qualified and recommended surgeons in your area. From among a small list, she should be able to schedule appointments, meet face to face, and make a decision based on *her* experience. Accompany her to these meetings. You will have an opinion as well.

Before your wife goes to these appointments, however, make sure she has all the pertinent information in hand or has her reports sent ahead to the doctor for review. Her pathology report, her breast scan and any medical information that will need to be considered should be in the surgeon's hands so that all cards are on the table. This way, you and the surgeon do not waste time rehashing the facts but can incorporate them with his opinions for a solution.

Moreover, make sure you and your wife come into each of these appointments with a list of questions. Write these down. Write down your concerns. Make certain your questions are answered, and be willing to listen closely.

If you are looking for a short list of questions that would be helpful in these appointments, begin with some of these:

- What procedure do you think would work best for my situation?

- Can you describe what you will do in this surgery?

- What will the prep and follow-up be like for this surgery?

- How often have you performed this surgery?

- How long will my recovery be?

- What additional doctors and staff will be involved in this procedure?

- Can you give me some of the pros and cons of this procedure, and what have other women experienced following this surgery?

- What are the odds that I will need chemo or radiation following this procedure?

- When will we know the results of the lymph node biopsy?

- What are the odds that I may develop lymphedema?

- What do you think would be important for me to know about this procedure?

- Are there any pamphlets or videos you could show me that might help me better understand how this procedure and recovery will work?

Of course, these are just suggested questions; your wife can create her own set. In fact, there may be other questions that will be far more important to her: questions about the surgeon's family (who is he/she?), experience or tenure, bedside manner (or how he treats his staff).

After a short time, there is no doubt that your wife will begin to form an opinion of the surgeon. Depending upon her prognosis and the type of cancer she has (slow or fast-growing, for example), she may gravitate to one surgeon over another. There are, of course, surgeons who specialize in various types of breast cancer, and your wife will want to seek out those surgeons who have strong reputations in the area of her diagnosis.

Although there is not much time to make the decision for a breast surgeon (or at least it can feel that way), a woman should be certain of her choice and work diligently to select the surgeon that is right for her. Some of this decision will be based on knowledge, and some on feeling. In fact, she might even say, "This surgeon just feels right for me."

Regardless, once you have made a choice, be confident. Doctors love the confidence of their patients. They thrive on it.

And then move on to the next decision.

The Oncologist/Radiation Oncologist

The oncologist is, in essence, the doctor in charge of treating your wife's cancer (if it has not been completely removed through surgery). Often a woman will not have to make a decision about the oncologist until after surgery, or as a secondary decision post-operative.

If post-operative treatment is required, the oncologist will become a familiar face. This physician will not only be meeting with your wife for those preliminary studies and treatment options, but he/she will be there for many follow-up conversations and through the entire corpus of treatments. A good oncologist is one who is thorough, insightful and available to answer questions through the treatments or even to provide support.

Many women discover that the post-operative treatments (chemo, especially) can be far more demanding than the surgery itself, so the oncologist she selects will need to be a trusted advisor and confidant. She may need an oncologist who can provide the latest and best that chemo or radiation treatment has to offer.

It never hurts to interview several oncologists before making a selection. I've known some women who have talked with half a dozen before making a selection. For some women, the oncologist may become the primary caregiver, so this is an important decision. Again, don't overlook the benefit of gathering information from other women who have been treated by a particular oncologist. You or your wife might discover some important facts and feelings about the oncologist based on the experiences of others. No doubt there will be many doctors in your area who would do a fantastic job.

Your wife's oncologist may, indeed, be the primary physician as far as she is concerned. And if your wife requires chemotherapy, she will likely have some initial conversation about this with the breast surgeon. In fact, the breast surgeon may work in cooperation with a partner who is an oncologist. So your wife may have a team approach from the beginning. Make sure you understand these relationships up front and take nothing for granted. Ask lots of questions. But if you and your wife are instructed to find your own oncologist, there will no doubt be some conversation with the breast surgeon at some point.

Again, because questions are helpful, here are some your wife may wish to take along to an initial appointment with an oncologist. These are only guidelines—suggestions, really—and so you will no doubt want to expand and formulate your own questions when you go to these appointments and strike up the banter.

- What type of cancer/tumor do I have, and how will you propose treating it?

- What can you tell me about my form of cancer and my treatment options?

- What are you recommending in my case, and why?

- How will these treatments affect me?

- What can you tell me about the results of my lymph node tests?

- What side effects might I experience?

- What are the risks with this treatment?

- What would you suggest that would help me re-main strong and confident through these treatments?

- How many treatments will there be, and how long will each treatment last?

- When will I begin treatment, and when will it end?

- How will these treatments impact me sexually, emotionally, or otherwise?

- What can you tell me about the odds of the cancer returning following these treatments?

- Could I, should I, be part of a study group?

- Are there any clinical trials I should be aware of?

- What final recommendations do you have for me?

Obviously, this is not a comprehensive list of questions, but rather a beginning point. Depending upon your oncologist and his/her personality and style, your wife will likely be given far more information than she can soak in at once, and so it never hurts to ponder the information for a few days. Other questions may emerge, and follow-up phone calls never hurt.

Every woman's cancer and needs are different, and you may be looking at chemo or radiation through a narrow lens. Chemo and radiation are also different in approach and focus (and even cancer type), so be aware that your wife may also want to know why one form of treatment is being considered over another. Women who go through radiation treatments will have a much different set of issues than those who go through chemotherapy. Keep this in mind, and be sure to explore all of these questions with the oncologists when you meet with them. As the caregiver, you can keep notes for your wife and be a second ear. Give attention to details, and help her retain some of the information the oncologist will be throwing at her.

Finally, allow your wife (or girlfriend, sister, mother, etc.) to be the judge of her own needs. You may have an opinion about an oncologist, but you should allow her to make this decision; this will play a big part in her "buy-in" and in her confidence in the treatments and their effectiveness. She will need to have a relationship built on confidence and trust. Support and encourage.

The Plastic Surgeon

Most men find this specialist's name a bit humorous. In fact, the plastic surgeon doesn't deal in plastic at all, but in human tissues. In the case of your wife, the plastic surgeon will be the one charged with restoring her breast(s), which many women associate with beauty, individuality, self-esteem, wholeness and sexuality. All of these things can be wrapped up in a woman's breast (and more), so you will want to be particularly sensitive and helpful when your wife talks to this surgeon.

However, you may also discover that the plastic surgeon is one of the most humorous doctors you will meet. He/she will likely have a good bedside manner—these doctors need to help patients feel good about themselves, especially after their bodies have been invaded by a scalpel. Plastic surgeons are usually very savvy when it comes to understanding a woman's feeling about her breast, and they usually interject a little humor to lighten the mood.

Plastic surgeons—in the case of lumpectomies and mastectomies—are doctors who restore the appearance and structure of the breast. This may involve tissue reconstruction, or in other cases, breast implants. Nipple reconstruction and "tattooing" may also be a part of this reconstruction process. Your wife will want to become familiar with every aspect of the plastic surgeon's recommendations and understand how the reconstruction surgeries will be accomplished, step by step.

The plastic surgeon may also invite the man to weigh in, too. I remember, when my wife was contemplating the breast reconstruction portion of her surgery and the plastic surgeon was discussing breast implants and showing us samples, the surgeon began demonstrating how he could "re-size" my wife. It was all very humorous at the time, and both of us appreciated the opportunity to consider how the reconstruction process would help restore my wife's body and appearance. Such things are important to women, and every woman has an opinion about what she will need as the final outcome for herself.

If your wife is going to receive a breast implant(s), she will also want to ask questions about the health risks, understand how a breast implant is inserted and maintained, and receive as much information as possible about that particular implant, such as how long it lasts and what it will feel like. Some women even want to feel the breasts of other women who have implants (my wife has offered a "feel" to other women who have questions about breast cancer and implants). Don't be surprised if your wife asks you to share your opinion or weigh in on the reconstruction process. She may believe that this part of the recovery journey will have a great impact on your relationship.

If you are looking for a short list of questions to ask your plastic surgeon, here are some suggestions to get you started:

- How will you reconstruct the breast?
- What steps are involved here, what are the side effects, and how long will it take for full recovery?
- In the case of implants, what do they feel like?
- How long does a typical implant last, and what happens if/when it needs to be replaced?
- What are the side effects of breast implants?
- Will other reconstruction be required, and what are my options here?
- What would you recommend in my case?

It is highly likely that your wife will want you to be present through all of these discussions with the plastic surgeon. Your support will mean a great deal to her, and it is one leg of the journey that you may actually share together in a more intimate way. You will be discussing things that will impact your future together and how your wife feels about herself. So don't be afraid to "kick the tires" and ask questions when you are in the plastic surgeon's office. You will learn a great deal about your wife through this process, and I am certain you will draw closer together.

Spiritual Help

Regardless of whether you and your wife are members of a church or synagogue, or whether you have a pastor, priest, rabbi or other spiritual guide in your life, don't overlook the spiritual dimensions of breast cancer recovery. If you have a pastor, for example, by all means inform this person of your need (pastors won't know unless you call) and invite him/her to offer presence and support, especially if a surgery is required or if there will be a long therapy afterward.

Many physicians (and even hospitals) will ask if you have a particular religious or spiritual affiliation and will offer to contact your spiritual leader. Even if you don't belong to a community of faith, most hospitals have chaplains who can offer prayer, support and comfort to both the patient and family.

Everyone, of course, has his/her own beliefs and spiritual path, and women who are faced with a breast cancer diagnosis will often begin to draw strength from these beliefs. Many physicians will also invite the pastor/chaplain to be present before the surgery, if the patient requests it.

Regardless of a patient's religious persuasion, there are also many resources available that can benefit the cancer patient spiritually. Many hospitals and clinics have racks of Care Notes ®. These brochures come in hundreds of titles, many of them dealing with topics that would be of interest to women and their families, who are making the journey through breast cancer. These Care Notes ® can also be found on line or ordered from the company's Web site. In addition, women and their families can find a wealth of spiritually directed books and first-person resources (such as *Chicken Soup for the Breast Cancer Survivor's Soul*). These books are not religious in nature but certainly contain much inspiration and spirit, which can assist in the breast cancer journey and keep motivation strong and positive. There are also breast cancer journals that can help women write their own reflections and engage in self-directed care, and these can be uplifting as well.

Another overlooked resource today is blogs. There are literally hundreds of breast cancer blogs out there written by women who are either in the midst of the journey or who are writing their thoughtd in retrospect. Many of these blogs can be very positive, and some will contain references to books, DVDs, journals and tips that can offer women and their families a wealth of spiritual help.

Many magazines, such as *Cure,* can provide women with the most up-to-date information about cancer and also provide inspirational stories in each issue. Subscriptions to *Cure* are free for cancer patients. There are many other magazines, online e-zines and journals that offer beautiful and positive reflections on the cancer journey.

So don't overlook the spiritual dimension of the healing process or the importance your own spirit and attitude will play in your wife's recovery. Men, in particular, may also benefit from talking to other men about how they coped with a wife's breast cancer diagnosis, and there can be a spiritual and healing component to these conversations. Don't be afraid to draw strength and support from those who can offer prayer, reflection or even a wider community of help.

Pre- and Post-Surgery Decisions

Selecting your medical team may be the biggest decisions you and your wife will make in the breast cancer journey. But there will be a myriad of smaller but no less weighty decisions that you will both make along the way.

Some of these decisions may involve adjusting work schedules or rearranging the bedroom and bath to make these spaces more conducive to recovery, or even deciding how the children will be cared for during a surgery or during the therapy sessions. Your wife may not feel like making many of these decisions, and so the bulk of them may come your way by default. Be prepared.

At the same time, don't forget to take care of yourself. If you, the caregiver, become tired or disinterested, then you will not be of value to your wife. Don't neglect keeping yourself in shape, eating right, or getting proper rest. Again, this may involve some re-arrangement of your schedule and time, but it will be worth it ... to both of you.

I will have to say that I felt more exhausted following my wife's surgery—after she came home to recover—than I did pre-surgery. I found that there was far more to do at home with the children, for example, and I also had to follow up with phone calls for insurance and the hospital. Much of this was time consuming and draining.

And then there is the fact that people call, or when they see you, they ask, "How is your wife doing?" They are, of course, concerned. But answering the same question over and over again can become deflating. Few people ask about the caregiver. Most don't ask, "How are *you* doing?"

I've known some men who became bitter in the post-operative world and who did not take care of themselves properly in the caregiver role. So, yes, it is vital that you stay positive, be aware of the many decisions and questions coming your way following surgery or treatment, and maintain a self-awareness and helpful attitude throughout.

Do not forget that you are helping your wife to regain a balance in her life—not just heal. You are a part of that balance. Even the smallest decisions you make at home can have a huge impact on her recovery.

₲ℛ

First Person

I was apprehensive about meeting the doctors who would be working on my wife. But it turned out to be nothing like I imagined. These meetings were not annual checkups, and so they spent more time with us detailing all of the fine points of the surgery and so forth. The oncologist my wife chose was super. I think he even called her at home one evening to see how she was feeling after her first week of chemo.

I remember that I had a long list of questions we wanted to ask. We had worked up the list at home, and then my wife wanted me to do most of the talking. It really wasn't my thing, but she thought she would forget what to ask. As it turns out, she did fine and actually ended up having good conversations and getting the answers she needed.

During my wife's mastectomy, there was a nurse who kept giving me updates. She kept asking me if I needed anything. That hospital seemed to have a special brand of caring.

I don't know if I have any particular insights for men, but I do think it helps when you can feel good about your surgeon and the people who are around you. There are some days when it is rather harrowing. Being able to talk to the doctor about a problem, or if you have a follow-up question, is important, too.

As it turns out, my wife came through the surgery very well, and after her treatments she has not had any reoccurrence. It's been seven years since she was released, and so we don't think about breast cancer as much as we used to. It kind of fades into the background. You get busy with life, doing other things, and eventually it all seems like it's ancient history.

Oh, and I might tell men to remember anniversaries. They can be important, too. It's important to remember being cancer free and all that you've been through together.

~Syd

ഇറ

Somebody who really helped me through this was our pastor. I don't know how people get through the rough places in life without faith or without a church family to support them. I think that would be very difficult.

Our pastor visited the day of my wife's surgery and had prayer with us, and—this really impressed me—our surgeon joined us in prayer, too. It was very comforting to know that we were appealing to God for help and healing.

I know most hospitals have chaplains, and I'm sure they would be glad to visit before or after the surgery. Yes, the pastor was very much a part of the team. I think faith played a large part in getting us through this. We are very thankful. God is good.

~Bill

Five Things to Remember

- You can help your wife assemble her "team," which may include a breast surgeon, an oncologist and a plastic surgeon.

- Help your wife do her homework and assemble a short list of doctors, and set up these appointments to get a feel for the best ones to treat the breast cancer.

- Assemble a list of questions before each appointment.

- Don't forget the spiritual aspect of healing.

- Be prepared to make other decisions pre- and post-surgery—many that may be unexpected.

Chapter Five
Family Matters

Breast cancer doesn't just impact an individual, it impacts the family, too. Women who receive a breast cancer diagnosis may be wives, mothers, grandmothers, sisters and aunts. Relationships are impacted. Family dynamics can change. And if there are children involved, one of the first questions you and your wife will ask is, "*What* do we tell the children, and *when* do we tell them?"

Naturally, a child's age determines how much he or she can understand of a situation, but in general it will be important that you talk about the breast cancer diagnosis with the family. Truth and accuracy will be important. Don't talk around cancer, veil the truth, or attempt to hide the upcoming surgery and/or treatments from the family. In fact, the family understanding and support will be critical to your wife's recovery and healing. The older your children are, for example, the more they can contribute and assist.

Having said this, however, it is important to realize that every family is different, and the way each person in the family reacts to a woman's breast cancer diagnosis will vary. If a family is aware and concerned for each other, then everyone will likely rally and find a supportive role in the journey. If there are marital struggles, or if the family is stressed for other reasons (such as financially), then an illness such as breast cancer can create even more stress.

The first step in the family journey can provide an opportunity to come together and find a new path. Everyone in the family can assume some portion of the burden, or—if one wants to create a positive spin—provide some service or help that could aid in the journey of healing.

Although our children were young when my wife was diagnosed with breast cancer, as parents we made a point of sharing the diagnosis with them early on, providing facts they could understand and answering questions as they emerged. Each of our children wanted to help Mom get better. We also prayed together, allowed the children to take on small tasks, and kept them informed of the major steps leading up to the surgery and the recovery at home. The children created cards for their mother, gave small gifts, and made a pledge that they would not worry and would do their best at school. As a husband and father I felt honored to be able to do all of these things—not only for my wife— but for the strength of the family. My wife was never alone through this ordeal, and she no doubt felt the support and love of her children. This love was a large factor in her recovery and healing.

It wasn't always easy for our children to understand what was happening, however. Sometimes they asked questions about their mother's absence at certain events at school, and I recall a few times when our son, the youngest, asked questions about death and was worried about his mother's illness. All of these were teaching moments—not always easy—and they provided another level of care and concern that was actually quite touching.

During this time, I recall talking to other husbands and dads whose wives were going through similar surgeries and treatments. It is amazing how, once you become part of the "breast cancer family," there is an amazing support network and bounty of relationships that emerge. I learned so much in a short period of time. There were men who told me, "My wife is a breast cancer survivor, too" or "my wife is going through treatments, also." In just a few weeks, I had a wealth of new friendships and information I had not expected.

Not all of our experiences and stories were the same, however. And family dynamics were different, too.

I recall talking to one man in our surgeon's waiting room who lamented his wife's breast cancer diagnosis as being not only unfortunate, but having "bad timing." Oddly enough, he confided that he didn't feel up to the task of being a caregiver, and he didn't want to disturb his teenage children's schedules by telling them about their mother's breast cancer. In fact, he approached it all as something of a family secret.

No doubt, breast cancer is a blow to any family, but a breast cancer diagnosis is not a death sentence. Men don't have to guard the secret or withhold information. Rather, being honest and forthright about the disease is most helpful and freeing. Withholding information from children may make them resentful later. They may question, later in their lives, the silence during their mother's illness.

In the event that you may need some tips for talking to your children about breast cancer, why not try a few of the following:

- **Do** give you and your wife some time to discuss the diagnosis together before you talk to your children. **Don't** go into a discussion with raw emotion, which can frighten younger children. Discuss how you will shape your words and when it is best to talk to the children soon after the diagnosis.

- **Do** remain as matter-of-fact and casual as you can in your conversation. Chances are, if you speak honestly, your children will soak in the realities and come to understand that, while breast cancer is a serious illness, it can be treated, and you are all going to help.

- **Do** talk to your doctor or care team about resources you can give to your children. There are many children's books for occasions such as this (see the bibliography).

- **Do** turn off the television, don't take phone calls, and put down the computers and cell phones when you begin talking about breast cancer. Don't allow interruptions to sidetrack your children's questions or your own thoughts.

- **Do** allow your children to ask questions. **Don't** tell your children that they shouldn't ask questions or feel sad or anxious.

- **Do** assure your children that their mother is going to get wonderful treatment and that all of these steps will help her to achieve the goal of getting well.

- **Do not** make promises you can't keep, such as telling the children that their mom will feel just fine by a certain date, or that she will attend an event, or even that things will soon be back to normal. Keep your guard up and keep the talk real.

- **Do** assure your children that they can help their mother, and invite them to think of some ways they would like to help. Form a plan, if you like, and even allow your children to write down some of their ideas.

- **Do** help your children to feel as though they are part of the solution—a part of the "team."

- **Do** assure your children of your love, in case you become emotional, and allow them to freely express their emotions, too.

- **Do** keep life as normal as possible for the children.

Through the journey of breast cancer, make it a point to stay as positive as possible. Stay positive not only in your outlook and approach, but also in your demeanor and your language. Be aware that you will need to be consistent in your positive approach, and rest assured that this attitude will impact your children daily. Children tend to emulate what they see in adults, and so staying upbeat may be the most important attitude you can exhibit.

Moms and Daughters

As a man, you might also be aware that moms and daughters can have a special bond through the breast cancer journey. The older the daughter—especially a teen—the greater the chances that she may have deeper concerns or even begin to ask personal questions about her own health or future. She might wonder, If Mom has breast cancer, will I get breast cancer, too? So the mother-daughter relationship is more complex in this situation. But you can help.

A few things that could be beneficial in this situation include:

- Allow your wife and daughter to have more time to talk about these issues.

- Invite your daughter to be a part of the consultation process or discussions with the doctors. Dr. Susan Love, in her excellent book *Dr. Susan Love's Breast Book*, indicates that many teenage girls have questions for the surgeon or desire to be a part of the consultation process. They might even have questions about their own genetic predisposition to breast cancer.

- Reassure your daughter that she is not alone in her fear and that you are also available to talk about these issues.

- Be aware that your daughter may need additional information about breast cancer (especially an older teen).

- Look for books and resources that might help your daughter (and Mom, too) navigate some of the deeper questions about the genetics of breast cancer.

Addressing Fears

If you have older children who are able to express their anxieties or ask deeper questions, don't be surprised if some of your conversations about breast cancer make their way to the dinner table or into other family time. Breast cancer can be frightening to children, and they may need reassurance, strength and answers to their questions. While you may not be able to answer every question, your willingness to talk about cancer can actually be one of the most important steps in alleviating their fears. Hiding the facts or refusing to speak about cancer can make it all the more frightening.

One of greatest fears children have—even if they don't speak of it—is "Will Mom die?" Naturally, people often equate cancer with death, and to a child or younger teen, the connection may seem obvious. But you can help alleviate these fears by speaking the truth—not sugarcoating—while also providing a balanced and logical answer. You can say something like, "We can expect Mom to live a very long time. Most women who have breast cancer have a full recovery, and there are doctors and nurses who are going to help Mom overcome the cancer."

Sometimes, when children's questions persist, it is helpful to have others outside of the immediate family help alleviate these fears. There may be someone in your family (a grandmother, aunt, or sister) who is also a breast cancer survivor. This person may be able to speak more personally and helpfully to a child and provide firsthand stories about breast cancer. Often, when a child can speak to someone who has already overcome a disease, she can see that it is not a death sentence. A child can see that there are others who have overcome breast cancer. They word "cancer" may not be so scary if other people can speak of it or even laugh about it.

As an aside to fears about death, some children also fear abandonment. They may see their mother, for example, leaving home more often for doctors' appointments and treatments, and they may not understand why Mom is not as readily available as before. They may not see the connection between these absences and the breast cancer.

Again, explanations can help, as can reassurance. If possible, try to engage your child's support in this healing process. Invite your child to help wherever possible, or to pray, or even to write letters of support when Mom is absent.

Some children may wonder how long the treatment and healing will take. They may not grasp the element of time very well (or even how short the healing process actually is!). From diagnosis to final treatment and eventually to normal life—these months can seem like years to a child. So some reassurance along the way never hurts.

Finally, two other fears that many children encounter take place after surgery. Some children are curious about Mom's scar (or reconstruction), while others may have a curiosity about a prosthesis (artificial breast) if Mom is wearing one.

Keep in mind that it is not necessary to show a scar to a child. Often an explanation of a "boo-boo" will suffice for younger children, and older children can grasp the concept. By the time the surgery is completed and Mom is home, there is already a sense of relief, and most children are happy enough to move on to other questions and concerns. If the next step in Mom's healing process is to undergo chemo or radiation treatments, these may become paramount.

In *Dr. Susan Love's Breast Book*, she relates a humorous story about a mother who chose to wear a prosthesis. Her children had questions about this artificial breast: what it looked like, what it was made of, how it was worn. The mother brought the prosthesis home, showed it to her children, and almost immediately they began treating it like a Frisbee, tossing it around the house. So much for fear and anxiety! Children are, indeed, resilient.

Regardless of your children's fears, the most important rule here is to be open and honest. Be willing to talk about these fears, and don't make them taboo or mysterious. Kids do have a remarkable capacity to grasp hope and embrace change.

Telling Your Extended Family

Soon after my wife was diagnosed with breast cancer, I recall having a conversation about our parents. My wife wondered, "When should I tell my parents about this?" and "How?"

A few thoughts here might help.

First, it is important to remember that one of the most compelling reasons to tell others about breast cancer is so we don't have to carry the burden alone. A support network is very important. Any time we can discuss a burden or anxiety with others, especially with those who love us, we discover a foundation of support.

Secondly, keep in mind that if you don't share the diagnosis and upcoming treatments with your extended family, they will likely find out the news from other sources and may feel slighted or hurt that you did not confide in them. We may not consider how quickly news spreads, especially if we have talked about the illness at all or even shared the news with close friends only. Word does travel fast, especially in this age of Facebook and iPhones. It doesn't take long for one person to drop word to another or for the grapevine of information to spread. News has never traveled faster than in our time, and distance is no longer a consideration.

Most doctors and oncologists will agree that it is best to tell others about the diagnosis earlier instead of later. If parents, grandparents or siblings are in the picture, don't hesitate to inform them about the breast cancer.

One of our friends, also a breast cancer survivor, described her feelings this way:

"I don't think that a cancer diagnosis should be a secret. At first I didn't want to tell my aging parents about my diagnosis because I thought it would upset them too much or cause them additional pain, but then I realized that I would be depriving them of the opportunity of caring about me. I didn't want to keep a secret. And, as it turned out, telling my parents about my breast cancer was one of the most freeing and helpful conversations. In fact, it was very hopeful."

So don't close up opportunities to tell your in-laws, siblings or parents about the diagnosis. Let others make the decision about how helpful or proactive they wish to be. In telling others about an illness, we are not necessarily asking for help; we are inviting them to be a part of the journey, in whatever ways they would like. Everyone (just like every family) is different, so people can make their own determinations about their degree of helpfulness.

In the event your spouse may be having a difficult time putting the words together to share with her parents or siblings, some suggestions here would be:

- Invite the family over to your house so you can relay the information together.

- If distance is an issue, make a phone call instead of relying on social media or text messages. We can't always relate our feelings through snippets of text.

- Don't overlook the possibility of using Skype or another video link to share with family who live far away.

- Use handwritten letters to relay deeper thoughts and express more heartfelt sentiments.

- Send materials (like brochures, pamphlets or booklets) that might better explain the procedures and treatments your spouse will be undertaking. Information never hurts, and it will also spare your family members from having to guess. They can learn more directly this way.

- Allow time and opportunity for the extended family to ask questions and affirm their willingness to help.

ഇന്ദ

First Person

My wife was diagnosed with breast cancer when she was forty-two, and I remember feeling at the time that we were being visited by an unwelcome guest. Breast cancer seemed like it was some kind of a numbers game—everyone was talking about the size of the tumor, the stages, if the numbers looked good, and so forth.

Our kids were young at the time: six, seven and ten, I think. But I don't recall ever feeling we were in it alone. At the time, my wife was very involved in organizing a preschool at the church, and there were many women who dropped by the house and brought casseroles and checked in on us. We never lacked for food. I do recall having conversations about diet, however, and we changed our food, trying to eat healthier.

The day of my wife's surgery was probably the most difficult for me, and it was really strange. Instead of going to the hospital, the doctor performed the lumpectomy in an outpatient clinic, and my wife wasn't even fully awake from the anesthesia yet when they told me I could take her home. I had driven our Astro van, and loading her into the front seat was quite an accomplishment.

Of course this was followed by weeks of radiation and chemo treatments. As I recall, I accompanied her to the appointments with the surgeon and the oncologist and to several of the treatments afterward.

My wife was incredible in her approach to this, especially getting the kids involved. When she started losing her hair, she asked the kids to shave her head. We had a shaving party, and they learned how to use the clippers. It wasn't a traumatic thing at all, but very supportive. My wife even timed some of her chemo appointments so she would be able to attend our daughter's wedding —which was a two-day drive from home. And later, when my wife was in Pittsburgh attending to her aunt's illness, I took the kids on a vacation to Disney World.

If there were any points of advice I would give to other men, I'd tell them to always be attentive to their wives' needs. Ask her what she wants. At least be available for every appointment, and let her know you are willing to sit with her.

If you have kids, I'd also advise keeping them involved. Even cancer can be a learning experience, although it's tough to know what kids are thinking. When kids are involved in taking care of Mom, they worry less and they are part of the healing, too.

I'd also advise people to be involved in a church. I can't say enough about how helpful people were in their support. It was tremendous. All the other Moms were helping out and bringing food.

I'm also amazed at how quickly my wife wanted to help other women as soon as her oncologist released her. She became one of those first-responders when other women were diagnosed with breast cancer. Along the way, all of our cancer anniversaries were significant. The first year, the second year. Being released from the doctor's annual checkup was a big one. There's a lot to celebrate.

Anyway, I'm a prostate cancer survivor, and I don't see anything among men that rivals the support and response that women bring to this. Whenever you hear "breast cancer," women come running to support. It's very inspiring.

~Don

Five Things to Remember:

- Remember that a breast cancer diagnosis impacts the whole family.

- If you have a daughter(s), a mother's breast cancer diagnosis will impact her differently. She will have other questions and concerns.

- Don't hide a breast cancer diagnosis from the family, especially not from children.

- By sharing the breast cancer diagnosis with the extended family, you will discover other levels of support, and much of this will be needed in the months ahead.

- Always be open and honest about your needs and your hopes for a full recovery.

Husband's Quick Guide to Money Management

Top 10 Things to Remember

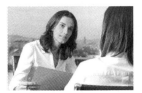

1. Call your insurance provider as early as possible.

2. Pre-plan, pre-register, prepare.

3. Don't hesitate to ask questions about fees, hospital costs, or costs of treatments.

4. If you get a second opinion, you may have a second set of financial figures to compare.

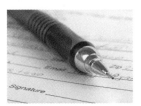

5. Don't forget to check your homeowners insurance policy if your wife is the principal breadwinner. Some policies may cover a portion of your mortgage payments in case your wife is incapacitated for a time.

6. If you have Medicare or Medicaid, review the covered costs of breast cancer care.

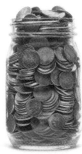

7. Always follow up with your insurance to make sure your costs were covered/ reimbursed per your policy.

8. Save as much as possible before surgery and treatment.

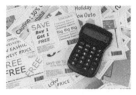

9. Cut out all unnecessary expenditures at home.

10. Now is the time to think about using some of your emergency fund. That's why you have saved it!

Chapter Six
Money Matters

In Woody Allen's slapstick comedy *Small Time Crooks*, we encounter a ragged married couple who are living from paycheck to paycheck. The husband, a bumbling dreamer played by Allen, hatches a plan for an elaborate bank heist that he believes will make them rich. His plan, of course, doesn't work, but as the couple is carrying out the heist they discover that his wife's talent for baking is their ticket to success. They do, indeed, become millionaires.

The success, however, is short-lived, as their marriage begins to tear apart at the very points where the money is holding them together. By the movie's end, we see the couple back where they started: penniless but deeply in love.

Although this is a comedy, the movie does portray some subtle truths about happiness in marriage and the role money does—or does not—play in creating it.

Breast cancer, of course, is no comedy, but in ways both apparent and subtle money enters into the picture. Many couples discover, for example, that a breast cancer diagnosis further heightens their awareness of money (or perhaps a lack of it or need for it), while others discover that money is merely a tool to help them address a problem—breast cancer.

A breast cancer diagnosis in and of itself cannot make or break a marriage, but financial concerns can certainly wrap some tight tentacles around a relationship and strangle it. There may be some men who will jump to this chapter of the book first, just to see how the finances are going to turn out or where they can turn for help. To be sure, having a clear picture of what a breast cancer diagnosis will mean financially can't hurt anyone, and in our contemporary climate of credit card debt, unemployment and foreclosure, adding one more financial log to the fire doesn't help.

But from the outset, remember: money won't make your marriage, but it won't necessarily help, either—not unless you have the proper outlook. That's what this chapter is about: providing a clearer picture of what will be involved from your bank account.

Exploring the "M" Word

Let's spend a little time talking about the "M" word as it relates to the "C" word. The truth is, no disease—and especially not breast cancer—is diagnosed and treated at the optimum time for anyone. In reality, you probably received this diagnosis and the subsequent billings for the surgery and treatment during the same week your mortgage, car and life insurance, utilities, Internet, taxes and credit card bills came due.

Well, if you are reading this book anticipating that money will somehow play into this equation for your family, you are probably right. Unless you have stellar health insurance, a wealthy aunt, or the means to write a check to cover all costs, you are probably going to feel some financial pinch along the way. Even with premier health insurance coverage, there are going to be intangible expenses you will pay out of pocket.

And let's face it; breast cancer can certainly turn a family upside down. A cancer diagnosis can place life on standstill and bring additional stress. Money is no different, and so it will be important to have a clear head about financial matters as you attempt to navigate the confusing and harrowing world of insurance, doctors and hospitals. You will likely hear a great deal of "Press 1 for more options" as you work through the insurance and health care system. Frustrations can mount. But if you are prepared, these money matters won't seem nearly as monumental.

Soon after my wife's diagnosis, I called my health insurance provider to get a clearer picture of the costs our family would be assuming for my wife's surgery and care. Even before the surgery, I had obtained information about our deductible and out-of-pocket expenses, as well as the peripheral costs, such as pain medication and pharmaceutical supplies. This information helped tremendously and gave us peace of mind as we approached the surgery date.

I also had an opportunity to talk to other men who were in the throes of navigating the health care system. Some of their stories were harrowing. Others were humorous. But after talking to many men about their own experiences, I have to say that I learned a great deal. There were many ideas offered, but here are three comments that were particularly helpful to me,and each provides an insight into the stressful world of managing money during a health crisis.

- "No one can be prepared for breast cancer, certainly not financially. But I learned that my insurance company wanted to be helpful, and it was imperative I find that one person inside the network whom I could talk to each time I had a question. If you can work with one person instead of many, it's a huge help."

- "When my wife was diagnosed with breast cancer, we didn't have health insurance. Financial worries were no doubt the biggest issues we faced following my wife's treatment. But I found a social worker who was able to help me navigate the hospital billing system, and they really worked with us."

- "Most important: keep all of your documents. Keep good records. Place them in a file for at least two years. You'll need these records more than you realize. Some of the bills are very slow in coming, and even the insurance company can get frustrated with the billing process. Don't worry over the records, but don't discard them."

Obviously, financial worries can add additional stress to the family, and some marriages can break under the strain. So don't think that you'll be able to navigate the breast cancer journey without discussing money. Eventually you will.

There are several tips that can help you in the financial arena. And there's so much you can learn from those who have walked this journey before you.

Insurance Insights

No doubt, by the time you read this book, health insurance will have changed—and perhaps changed again—and so the first thing you'll need to know about insurance is to *know your insurance*. Find your policy, read it closely, make sure you understand all the finer points and how your policy will work. Make sure you know what your deductible is and what it covers. Call your insurance agent and begin working with someone "inside" who can answer questions for you when they arise. Try to get a direct line to this person so you can call back when you have a need. Consistency will be of paramount importance in the days ahead.

Be certain you also understand all of the preapproval requirements and procedures and follow them explicitly so you will not be caught in a loophole. In addition, be certain to ask questions about follow-up surgeries such as reconstruction (breast implants, etc.) and even nipple reconstruction and tattooing. Some insurance companies want to treat these secondary procedures as optional or cosmetic, so it will be imperative that you clarify what is and is not covered under your plan. Clarity can go a long way to giving you peace of mind, and it will also help you plan for these procedures in case they are not included in your health plan.

No doubt, for most men, the insurance labyrinth can be one of the most frustrating and harrowing parts of the breast cancer experience. We can handle the housework and the additional strain of cooking and carting the children, but an HMO is another matter. Often, it is difficult to get answers—even from top health care providers—and the amount of time that can be spent on the telephone or on the Internet can be staggering. Frustrations can mount. So tread lightly on your insurance experience and go into it with a level head and carefully detailed set of questions. Write down what you need to know, what you want to ask. Have this in front of you each time you talk, and write down the answers you are given. Don't assume your memory will hold. Keep good records.

As far as insurance is concerned, here are ten tips that will land you in good stead.

- Begin with a clear understanding of your preapproval requirements for the hospital and all surgeries and outpatient follow-ups.

- Understand the guidelines for obtaining a second (or even third) opinion from a surgeon or specialist.

- Understand the procedures required for filing claims.

- Obtain copies of all claims and the various forms.

- Know what your deductible is and how it applies to the full range of your wife's treatment and care from beginning to end, as well as into, potentially, a second "year" of coverage.

- Understand any limits imposed on surgery, treatments and other procedures that are part of the breast cancer diagnosis.

- Understand if your policy covers any "new" or "alternative" procedures. Since procedures and treatment options are continually adapting, it will be interesting and useful to know what your insurance provider considers traditional or alternative.

- Be certain to ask about the reconstructive phase and breast restoration. Again, most plans will cover this and will not consider it "optional," but clarity is always best.

- Create a filing system for all of the documents you will receive (bills, etc.) from the hospital, breast surgeon, visits, plastic surgeon, pharmacy, etc.

- Keep good records, make copies, and don't discard anything for at least two years following the final billing. Sometimes late bills arrive and the system can be extremely slow.

In addition to these tips for handling your insurance, you may also benefit by keeping the following records to help you navigate the various appointments and procedures in the months ahead.

- Keep a calendar (create a file on your smart phone or computer) of all appointments.

- Inside this calendar keep a record of all medications, as well as the times they are to be administered, and recovery steps given by the doctors.

- Always bring claim forms with you to the doctors, if required, and create a travel file that you can pick up easily and handily. You don't want to have to search for these important papers every time you have an appointment.

- Always ask that a copy of the billings be sent to you as well as your insurance company.

- Check in with your insurance provider periodically to make sure payments are being made.

- Gather the names of the people you should talk to in, for example, your surgeon's office. Having a list of "go to" people will save you time and energy if you do have a question down the road. Whenever possible, obtain a direct phone number to this person who can help you.

- Make certain you are keeping all of your insurance premiums (payments) up to date. In the thick of worrying about paying other bills, don't forget to pay your insurance premiums!

Again, don't think that you are the first man who has ever shouldered a financial burden when it comes to an unexpected disease or diagnosis. Others have walked in your shoes. Seek out others who can help you if you are having financial worries or even emotional struggles. Financial worries can often be the most unsettling and the most harrowing, so don't allow these frustrations to bottleneck inside of you.

Getting Help

Because breast cancer can be diagnosed in women who are younger or older, there is no one answer for couples who are experiencing a financial burden. For older couples, Medicare (and sometimes Medicaid) can assist in, or even alleviate, the financial needs of a surgery and treatment. For younger couples, a good health insurance policy can be key.

But what if these resources are not available? What if a couple has no health insurance (due to unemployment, disability, etc.)?

In the latter case, it will be important to discuss your situation at the outset with the hospital, surgeon and other medical staff involved. Many hospitals will set up payment plans, and likewise some doctors will work with patients and their families to create a feasible payment plan.

Naturally, if a couple has an emergency fund for needs such as this, it is a great thing. But not all emergency funds can cover the costs of surgery and treatment. Sometimes, other forms of assistance are needed.

Be aware that most hospitals have social workers who can assist with financial needs or serve as a liaison with the hospital. Likewise, there are breast cancer support groups and nonprofit organizations in your area that might be able to give you certain kinds of assistance.

Check out some of the organizations noted in the back of this book, and peruse the various Web sites. Write for information. Most of these organizations also have hotlines or forums where people can ask questions. Don't be afraid to reach out for other solutions and answers if you find yourself in a financial bind.

The answers might not always be easy or forthcoming, but if you continue to look for a solution, you can often discover resources and ways to meet the need. Again, you are not alone in this struggle, and you should not hesitate to use the large national breast cancer organizations to obtain information about creative solutions.

Financial Fallout

While it is not true for every family, finances can often prove problematic during and after a breast cancer diagnosis, especially when it comes to marriages. As one friend of mine recently noted, breast cancer has a tendency to create emotional and relational difficulties. A diagnosis is difficult enough without financial fallout, but if money is a problem, marital discord can often be exposed.

Although my wife's diagnosis did not threaten an end to our marriage— in fact, it drew us closer together—I do recall that financial worries were ever on my mind. And since I was the one who was attempting to keep records and stay on top of the insurance claims, it often felt like I was carrying an additional burden. Sometimes it seemed unfair.

In the meantime, my wife was going through changes of her own. Like most women who are diagnosed with breast cancer, my wife began a process of soul-searching that led her, eventually, onto a new career path. Soon after her recovery, she told me she wanted to go back to school, earn a second degree in science, and become a teacher. She wanted to leave behind the world of pharmaceutical sales and pursue a dream of helping teenagers.

Not all women make these types of drastic changes in their careers, but it is not uncommon for women to begin thinking about the trajectory of their lives and to dream new dreams. Some of this may be due to our own feelings of mortality. Or sometimes a serious illness shocks our thinking and sets us on another path. The new post-cancer path can also be an additional expense. As in our case, when my wife went back to school, we lost that second income (and she was the primary breadwinner to boot). Naturally, our financial picture changed remarkably post-cancer. So we had to make changes to our lifestyle and spending habits (even our needs).

Breast cancer can also be expensive in ways other than paying deductibles and pharmaceutical bills. Many women, following their recovery, need therapy of another kind. They may feel a need to purchase new clothing or undergarments, especially if they are self-conscious about their appearance or think they look different. Indeed, some women will lose weight through the ordeal, while others might gain, so an adjustment in self-image is typical.

Often breast cancer survivors need to pamper themselves with some new attire or perhaps a new hairstyle, or they may even desire to drive something different.

In my wife's case, she decided she wanted to learn how to ride a motorcycle. But I have also known women who felt more confident in a new car or with a new job, or even decided to take up a new hobby. All of this is to say that breast cancer survivors do see every day as a gift, and there may be a new outlook that compels them to want to do more or experience more. Some of these endeavors may cost a few dollars, so it is best to be prepared for these realities.

Other women worry about employment following breast cancer treatment. They wonder if their employer will keep them on the plan or will hold their jobs for them during the surgery and recovery period (which can, after all, be quite lengthy). These are not easy questions to answer, and unfortunately some women do experience discrimination in this way.

However, current laws are set up that prohibit employers from dismissing on the basis of breast cancer treatment, and women should not feel threatened. Discussing the reality early with the employer is a key thing, and most women end up receiving a great deal of support from their network of friends at their workplace. So, while employment may be a concern at first, you should feel assured that any decent employer should be willing to demonstrate support before, during and after the surgery. These realities are part of the health landscape now.

I note these things in no small part because many marriages do suffer soon after recovery from breast cancer. And for many couples, financial stresses can be at the center of these concerns. Many couples struggle to find solutions to these stresses, and not all marriages survive the fallout.

What can you do to insure that you stay strong in *your* relationship?

Here are a few tips that might help.

First, make sure you communicate effectively and honestly with your spouse. Don't forget: good communication involves both speaking *and* listening. So be a good listener. If you pick up on concerns that your wife is having, be willing to listen to her and do not withdraw.

Secondly, affirm your wife's feelings if she is experiencing a sense of restlessness or a need to change. Certainly, we all value stability in life, and we all need those aspects of life that we can count on. But there is also a part of us that values a new, fresh approach. Often breast cancer intensifies these feelings in a woman, and some may express a desire to change, whether it be their career or even their location. Keep in mind that you can help your wife as she sorts through these feelings by affirming her value, her worth, her importance.

Finally, even if you are experiencing financial difficulties through the breast cancer journey, don't forget to take care of each other. Keep in mind that you are also fighting the battle *together*. Plan simple times together. Go to a movie. Take a walk. Take a weekend trip. Your time together doesn't have to be an additional financial burden, and you can be learning how to manage breast cancer without allowing it to overcome your relationship. Even a small gift can go a long way in making your wife feel appreciated and valued.

So ... don't let finances be the ruin of your relationship. Remember, you will have time in the future to attend to these financial needs, but you will need your wife!

Finances may not be an issue for many couples, but even the savviest and most financially astute will discover that breast cancer offers a new twist to the relationship. Even though money may not be the most important factor, be aware of your financial picture as you journey through cancer together.

₞ℓℲ

First Person

My wife was diagnosed with breast cancer at a fairly young age—before her fortieth birthday. So we were not prepared for this news at all. It was a jolt.

Having younger children, our life was centered around homework, school functions and weekend trips to Grandma's house. But all of that changed. Suddenly we were tossed into this world of biopsy and surgery. We had to weigh our options quickly, and in the end my wife opted to have a bilateral mastectomy. She just didn't want to worry about a recurrence in the other breast and wanted to feel like she could get on with her life.

This was difficult for me, of course, but I wanted to support whatever she felt was best for her health.

We had a lot of questions, though, about finances. We knew we would have to put some things on hold for a while. I had good insurance through my work, but it was still tough trying to figure out all of the paperwork and making all of the phone calls. Our biggest worries up to this point were paying the mortgage and the car, maybe saving a few dollars when we could for future college educations. We did take some nice vacations. Overall, though, it worked out better than I imagined, and we didn't end up with staggering bills. It was all manageable. We cut back on some trips and things like that, but we didn't mind, since the cancer sort of changed how we were approaching life, anyway.

You know, things get a lot simpler after cancer. I think you see life differently. My wife does, certainly. But I do, too. We don't have to have the best cars, the best vacations, the best meals anymore. Now it's about making more time for each other and spending more time as a family. You know ... simple pursuits. We really made an attempt to keep our lives simple after the cancer, and I think this has been one of the biggest changes we've experienced. We didn't get caught up in pursing the wrong things.

Anyway, I wouldn't say that cancer was a blessing (who would say that?), but I do know that breast cancer changed our lives. We had to grow in ways we would not have grown otherwise. And we've been able to help some of our friends and family now who are going through similar circumstances. It's amazing how many people you meet who are going through the same thing. So this has been remarkable, too. Being able to help other people. I actually enjoy talking to other men about the experience. It makes me realize how fortunate we are that my wife is completely cured of this disease and she doesn't have to worry about a recurrence.

If I had one piece of advice for other men it would be—don't worry. This may sound strange, and I know it's difficult to do, but worry doesn't solve anything. Let the doctors and specialists do their jobs. The knowledge and treatments available these days is tremendous. I'm impressed. The best thing a man can do is be strong in his support and attend to all of the details so she can focus on getting well.

It worked for me.

~James

Five Things to Remember:

- Speak to your health insurance provider about your deductible, your coverage and the procedures that will be involved.

- Organize and keep a file of all paperwork, as you will need these records months down the road.

- If you need financial help, work with the hospital and other organizations to get answers.

- Communicate with your spouse about your financial picture.

- Regardless of your financial picture, make time for each other and keep your marriage strong.

Husband's Quick Guide to Family Care

Top 10 Things to Remember

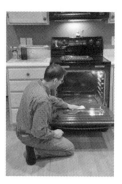

1. A breast cancer diagnosis will impact the entire family, including the children.

2. Your wife may be preoccupied with her health and treatment decisions and may lean more heavily upon you to be caregiver, chef and parent.

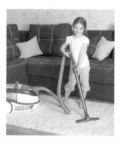

3. Explain to children what is happening using age-appropriate information and language.

4. Always tell the truth and answer questions that older children will have.

5. As the children can, and desire, allow them to help in your wife's support and healing.

6. There may be other family members (parents and siblings) who can be vital caregivers and helpers during the breast cancer journey.

7. Allow other family members to help as they can.

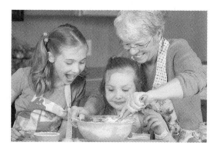

8. Be aware that a breast cancer diagnosis will impact your marriage in some ways (but may strengthen your relationship if you allow it).

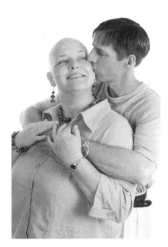

9. Be a positive force for the family during your breast cancer journey.

10. Take care of yourself so you can take care of others.

Chapter Seven
The Road to Recovery

Earlier you read about ways you could be helpful to your wife during the recovery phase. Now we'll delve a bit deeper into the post-surgery experience.

Keep in mind that every woman's recovery (treatments, pace, relational, etc.) will be different. Some women may be recovering from a mastectomy but will not be taking radiation or chemotherapy. Other women may have opted for a lumpectomy followed by radiation. Others may be engaged in a longer treatment program centered around both radiation and chemo, or perhaps even a follow-up surgery. The road can be short or long. It can have obstacles, even pitfalls. There can be detours and roundabouts and expressways.

Part of your role will be keeping your wife positive, motivated and moving toward the goal. The majority of women recover fully from breast cancer, and keeping this end in mind can be one of your most important tasks.

Many women grow tired at some point along the way, and your energy can be vital to your wife's outlook. Both of you will need perseverance and hope. It is a cliché, but it is important to take one day at a time.

Having talked to many breast cancer survivors, it seems that setting short-term goals can be most helpful. Looking too far down the road and becoming overly burdened by all the steps of surgery, reconstruction, radiation or chemo is much too heavy. Break down the recovery process into phases or steps. Remind your wife daily that she is doing well and that all she needs to focus on is the next step, the next day. Attempting to tackle too much too soon (emotionally and intellectually) is usually counterproductive. Be her advocate. Be her cheerleader. Be her friend.

If your wife does have several steps in the recovery process, it is helpful to understand each one. So, let's have a deeper look at the various forms of treatment in recovery and what these might mean for your wife.

Post-Surgery

Whether your wife opted for a lumpectomy and radiation or a single or double mastectomy, there is going to be post-surgery recovery. This time will be defined by discomfort, pain, anxiety and exercises (stretching and strength). Your wife should also expect fatigue and, perhaps, an inability to sleep comfortably or soundly. She may also have some nausea, but this should not be a carry-over from the anesthesia. Check with the doctor if the nausea persists.

The stretching movements that the doctor has assigned will be particularly important to her recovery. Not only will exercises give her more energy and help her body to produce hormones and process nutrition, but they will be essential to her flexibility in the years ahead. Some women develop stiff shoulders or joints following surgery and may also feel somewhat inhibited by a breast implant. However, following the regimen—especially through the pain—will reduce her risk of developing this long-term stiffness. Again, a cliché, but no pain means no gain. Help her manage her discomfort by urging her on. Be her coach.

Also, ask your doctor about other exercise options. If your wife is into fitness before her surgery, she may appreciate participating in a YMCA program, for instance. There may also be classes in your area specifically designed for surgery recovery. Some of these nonimpact programs are excellent and can provide a group dynamic and inspiration she may not be able to find at home.

Be aware that your wife may also worry about her scar. Make sure she continues to apply the various ointments and antibiotic medications, and remind her that the brightness of the scar will fade over time. You may also note changes, day by day, that she does not see in the mirror. These gentle reminders can be helpful. Some incisions may take a year to heal completely, so don't rush the healing process, either.

The incision may also continue to be a source of pain for your wife in the months ahead. Remember, her body has been invaded, and in a very sensitive area of the body. According to Dr. Susan Love, nearly half of all women say they experience some form of pain (whether "shooting," "stabbing" or "tiring") in the surgically repaired breast months after surgery. So the post-recovery process is not necessarily quick.

The post-surgery period can also be described as a period of physical adjustment. You and your wife may develop new sleeping patterns, eating patterns or work habits. You may also rediscover your sexual chemistry. Your wife may need different sexual expressions from you, and some of your old patterns of foreplay or lovemaking may not work as well in the post-surgery bedroom. You may need to talk about these things, and perhaps you will discover that your communication and intimacy has deepened because of it.

Consider the first year after surgery as a period of adjustment. Take nothing for granted. And if you ever feel you need help from the physicians, or even if you have questions about certain aspects of the healing process or pain levels, don't hesitate to contact them.

In the end, your consistency will be one of the most influential factors in your wife's recovery. The more you know, the more you can help. And the more you help, the faster your wife will heal.

Radiation Therapy

As noted above, radiation therapy is most commonly applied in conjunction with a lumpectomy, but it can also be used as a local control when a tumor is found in a certain area of the body. Women selecting this option believe it is the *best for them* (and so, for them, it is!).

Radiation therapists can explain the techniques and philosophy of radiation therapy in a more complete way, but a thumbnail sketch of the technique is essentially as follows:

- Each weekday (Monday-Friday) a certain amount of radiation (measured in rads) is applied to an area of the affected breast.
- This treatment continues for some weeks (usually six).

For most women, the side effects and weakness associated with radiation are less than that of chemotherapy. However, radiation therapy can make some women nauseous, weak, or affect changes in the skin and breast tissue (where a hardness can develop).

Keep in mind that, for most women who opt for a lumpectomy and radiation, they can resume work and their usual daily schedule as soon as they have rested and healed from the surgery. So radiation is the kind of treatment that can be scheduled around the woman's preferences.

One couple I know used to argue about the radiation schedule. The husband was adamant that his wife should receive the daily treatment after work, when she had finished with her day and would be prepared to come home and rest. But this never appealed to her. Rather, she preferred the early morning schedule and ended up stopping in for her dose of radiation on the way to work. She explained, "I didn't want to have the radiation hanging over my head all day, thinking about it. I wanted to get it out of the way first thing, so I could resume my normal life. I was probably more tired at work, but then at home I could rest and prepare myself for the next day."

Naturally, she won the argument. And every woman who receives a daily dose of radiation will have a preferred time of day. It's her life, and she will need to make the decision based on her own energy and focus. Give her your support.

Radiation, as noted above, is not without other side effects. Some women may feel a tenderness in the breast, or under the arm, or even in the cheeks or throat. In certain cases, some women may also develop a burned appearance in the breast or under the arm. These cases, especially, can be more painful, but salves and ointments are available to soothe the affected areas. Men may wonder whether they should go to every radiation appointment with their wife. Short answer: no (Unless she wants you to!) But if you are going to be supportive, you will want to accompany her for the initial treatments so you can meet the doctors, the nurses and the staff who will be administering the treatments. This is a nice touch, and the caregivers and your wife will thank you for it.

One other factor in radiation is the need for patience. Radiation is a long haul (usually six weeks), and many women and their husbands describe the radiation schedule as "grueling" or "interminable." It is long. But one of the keys is to stay engaged in life—to focus on your blessings and the things you enjoy. On the days when your wife does not have radiation, make a point to do something special or get extra rest if she needs the recuperation. You can almost make marks on the calendar and begin checking them off as you go along. Day by day. Week by week. Think of those weeks as you would the innings of a baseball game. Eventually you'll find yourself in the seventh-inning stretch, and one day you'll be in the bottom of the ninth.

When your wife comes home from radiation for the last time, be sure to have a celebration. Just don't light any candles. Think ice cream and cake instead.

Chemotherapy

The world of chemotherapy will vary from woman to woman. And chemo itself also varies in form, style and amount based on the type of cancer and the treatment designated. Some women will opt to continue to work during the weeks of chemo treatment, while others may want to scale back in the workplace or take a leave of absence.

These options are something you should discuss, and your doctor may be able to provide insights based on the energy level and responses of other patients to the respective chemo. Some types of chemo have a tendency to produce more nausea. Others not. And every woman is different in terms of her energy and response to the treatments.

One of the men I interviewed explained it this way:

"My wife was always resilient in the face of her chemo treatments, but I could tell that, as the weeks went by, it was starting to wear her down. She was working her full schedule when she started the treatments, but as the weeks wore on and she began to lose her hair, she didn't feel the same compulsion to go to work. That's when she asked for a leave of absence so she could focus on the battle. She also wanted to be at home and not have to worry about her appearance. She did find a

wig she liked, but she didn't particularly like wearing it. So the decision to essentially focus full time on completing the chemo was a big step for her. And it was for me, too." (Tom)

Women who are taking chemo can benefit from some basic guidance from those who have walked the chemo walk. After talking to several women who have undergone chemo, I learned that they each had something to offer by way of advice. A few points for women:

- Nausea seems to be the most difficult side effect, but they can reduce the severity of it by staying away from movement. Even riding an excessive amount in a car or having a long drive to and from the chemo treatments can bring on the feeling. She should rest as much as possible.

- Sometimes the anti-nausea bands (used most commonly on cruises) or an over-the-counter motion sickness pill can do the trick.

- Sometimes a ginger candy, or even the scent of ginger, can be an anti-nausea medication.

- Going on short walks during the chemo period can help keep the body strong. Nothing strenuous, mind you, but stretching and flexibility can actually make the chemo treatments less stressful on the body.

- Having a wig picked out before the treatments begin can be therapeutic. Doing this before your wife is tired and washed out can also save her from worry and anxiety.

- If your wife is planning to go back to work, make sure she understands her employer's policies regarding medical leave, and, if possible, alerts her employer to her chemo schedule. People in companies have hearts, too, and she may discover more support from her company than she expects.

- Make sure you—or a friend or family member—can drive your wife to and from the chemo treatments, especially as they wear into weeks. Some women begin the treatments on their own, only to discover they are getting too tired or don't have the focus to drive themselves home. Be sure she has someone lined up to help when she might need it.

- A woman should not feel that she can do all of this on her own. It is acceptable to ask for assistance. She may not feel like cooking, or even eating, for some time. Some smells may make her nauseated, too. So she shouldn't be afraid to let you know what she needs.

As you can see, chemo is not for the faint of heart. Your wife will need to have resolve to finish strong. And you will need to be ready to assist in everything from driving to cooking to gentle reminders. You may especially need to help her if she begins to lose her hair. This can be traumatic, even though women will be prepared for it intellectually. Your love, your affirmation and your reminders that she is beautiful will be most important to her.

Some men told me they made it a point to accompany their wives to each chemo treatment. Others allowed their wives to go alone or with a friend, then offered support at home. Make certain you understand your wife's preference. It wouldn't do—*and the two of you wouldn't do well*—if she was expecting you to be present, but you opted out for work or a game of golf.

Chemo rooms are never pleasant places to visit. The wait during the treatment itself is often described as the most stressful part of the experience. While the staff at the center will certainly do their best to keep you positive and engaged, it may be up to you to give your wife an emotional lift. As time goes by, she may dread the experience. You can encourage her along and help her to realize that she is making progress, that you are engaged in the cancer battle together. She is not alone in the fight.

Keep in mind that certain kinds of chemo treatments can be lengthy. It is not uncommon to sit in the chemo room for an hour, or even two. So you may want to bring along some good reading material (your wife, too) or perhaps have some engaging conversation. Don't focus on problems at home, however, or

119

discuss difficulties with your children or your work. Make sure you don't add stress to your wife's experience, and if she gets off on a negative or cynical tangent, reign her back with a joke or an insight that is uplifting. Be prepared for *anything*, and be aware of *everything*.

Back on the home front, make sure your wife drinks plenty of water during her chemo cycle, and be aware that she may not always feel like eating what she has always enjoyed. In fact, she may not want to risk disliking a favorite food, so you may want to ask her about the meals. Most women do well with more basic foods. Nothing fancy. Just keep her water glass filled and create the kind of food she feels she can tolerate.

If you have children, make them aware that their mother is going through a tedious process of healing, and remind them that Mom can use their help. They will probably enjoy giving her nice gifts, making encouraging cards, or writing letters. You can also invite her friends and co-workers to send their greetings, too. It's all good. And this love and friendship will give her a boost on those days when she is feeling particularly weary or low.

Finally, when it comes to chemo, don't take your wife's emotions so personally. Keep in mind that there may be some days when she will be angry, short-tempered, or tired. Give her a break on these bad days, and rest assured that if your wife has a sweet disposition or a soft temperament, it will return soon after the treatments are complete. Don't respond to any curt comments or angry tone. Assure her that you understand and will do all you can to give her the proper rest and energy she needs. Remember, your emotions are also being interjected into the mix, just like the chemo itself, so any emotion you are putting out will also be added to the experience.

As you go through this chemo journey together, rest assured it will soon come to an end. All troubling things do. They say that nothing good ever lasts, but if that's true, it certainly holds for the bad experiences, as well. One day you will be chemo-free. And cancer-free, as well.

Look forward to that day, that good word. And then you can look back on the days of chemotherapy with something akin to a smile and say together: we beat it!

Hormone Therapy

There are a variety of opinions about hormone replacement therapy (HRT), both in term of benefits and risks. In fact, the more I read about it, the more confused I am. Perhaps your wife has been reading about the benefits and risks of this post-cancer therapy or has even studied it as a cancer preventative. Again, physicians and clinical experts seem divided, and there is mounting data being gathered on a variety of fronts. Tamoxifen is probably one of the most talked about estrogen blockers of the past decade.

Any discussion of hormone replacement therapy should be conducted with your doctor's input (and probably secondary opinions also). Keep in mind that, as with most therapies, one can probably find a doctor who will support or discourage it based on his/her experience or background, so multiple opinions will be more informative.

Obviously HRT has its place in the arsenal of treatments; otherwise it would not be an option. And as with any other treatment, women benefit most by doing their own research, talking to as many doctors as possible, and then making the informed decision that she thinks is right for her. There are ample books and articles out there—and far more on the Internet than one can possible read—pertaining to Tamoxifen and other HRT options. Keep reading. Keep asking. And eventually you and your wife will arrive at the juncture where information and personal needs meet.

Better yet, talk to some women who have actually used HRT pre- or post-cancer. They will be able to tell you a great deal about what it is, what it does, and how it worked for them.

Recovering Your Sex Life

Many men want to know: "When does sex return after surgery?"

Answers vary from couple to couple, of course. What may be torrid sexual activity and frequency to one couple may seem sporadic to another. But there are some basic (if not common sense) realities that can guide any man through his questions.

First, few women are going to feel "sexy" or desirable hours after surgery, whether after a lumpectomy or mastectomy. There is also going to be some level of pain. So guys should be aware that while women may crave touch and tenderness, this may not be a prelude to sexual activity. Holding, kissing and caressing will be important for most women. And post-surgery is also a time for men to discover how to be more "in touch" with their wives on levels other than sexual.

As the pain from surgery subsides, some women may feel sexy again or even desire sex, but there will still be a need for gentleness and, perhaps, some awkward positioning in the weeks immediately after a mastectomy. Keep in mind that a woman after surgery is not going to be able to move her arms without some discomfort, and there may be many positions that are simply awkward at best or painful at their worst. If sex is desired, make sure your wife is getting what she needs and is comfortable throughout. Easy does it. And just use common sense.

When a woman is taking radiation therapy, she may find that she has more energy at the beginning of these treatments than she does toward the end. So time and timing are again a factor in libido. Women taking radiation may also have more energy in the mornings (or prior to a treatment), so creating these times to be together may also be a matter of planning and dating. Sex may not be so spontaneous during radiation, but couples can always plan for intimacy during the best days.

Chemotherapy offers other challenges to one's sex life. Many doctors will discourage intercourse or oral sex in the hours immediately following a chemo treatment, as the vaginal walls can secrete some of the chemo drug. Condoms could be used, but then the vaginal walls may also be tender or dry during this period of chemotherapy, and couples should plan accordingly. Having a lubricant at the bedside can be a good idea during the weeks of chemotherapy or even the months afterward.

It would be a stretch to say that every couple's sex life returns to its previous level following the days of surgery (and/or therapy). Many couples need to rediscover their sexual identity again. And so it is not a bad idea to plan some special romantic weekends or, perhaps, a type of second honeymoon, in order to recapture some of the intimacy and sexual spark. Make plans to spice up your sexual repertoire. Wait until after your wife has fully recovered and is regaining her strength and vibrancy again to plan these times. But do plan them.

Then there are those couples who maintain that their sex lives actually improve following the cancer experience. Finding a new level of intimacy battling cancer together can certainly be a factor. Intimacy is far more than sex. Intimacy actually involves vulnerability, honesty, openness, self-expression and commitment to the other's needs. When couples find this—and many do discover it through the cancer journey—there is a new urgency and meaning in sex that was not there before. Sex takes on a deeper importance and a new kind of "oneness" that can be traced to this newfound intimacy.

I'm not sure that my own sex life improved after my wife's mastectomy, but I know my love for her deepened, and it has continued to deepen in the years afterward. Some of this feeds back to the cancer journey we shared together. And I know that our levels of intimacy have continued to deepen as we have grown older together. Sex means a lot more to us now than it did when we were in our twenties. I'm not thankful for cancer, but I am grateful for each day we share together and for what we have accomplished through the enormous challenges of illness, parenting and dual careers post-cancer.

I know I'm not the only man who has experienced this. Many cancer survivors share similar experiences of deepening sexual intimacy because of the newfound togetherness.

Post-cancer, I also began writing love/romance poetry to my wife (usually weekly), and I've had a great many of these poems published. I'm always amazed that editors find my poems desirable for a wider audience, but I guess that's what comes from writing honestly and from the heart. My wife hasn't read most of these poems—sometimes she only sees them after they are published. And a great many of my private poems are silly (some may be categorized as erotic, bawdy or warped), but others hearken back to the cancer experience, and through these poems I hope to offer insights about the cancer experience to others. Here's a sonnet about breast implants, for example, that many people have appreciated.

123

Breast Implants

The plastic surgeon seems to enjoy his work:
Holding the jelly orbs in his capable hands
And telling my wife that after her surgery
He will recreate what the cancer has taken.
How strange these are, jiggling in the light,
esembling nothing I have cupped or kissed,
Hoping that after our world has been shaken
There is restoration in his expertise.

My wife selects her breast like a used car—
Testing the various models for their heft
And warming to the touch of one. We are
Happy with the choice and sign the line.
We trust there will be life in what is left,
And after silicone, more time.

The final point I would like to make in regard to sex is this: if you are worried about your sex life following breast cancer, you can do a great deal during your wife's recovery period to light the fire again, or at least keep the embers smoldering. As any psychologist or sex therapist will attest, if a man is attending to his wife's needs, helping out around the house, showering her with love and attention, and is open and honest about his feelings, he's going to get a passionate response when his wife feels better. Heck, he may get more than he bargained for or may have more demand than he can meet.

And keep in mind that, all things considered, your wife's recovery period—even if it involves radiation, chemo or both—is a rather short span of time in the scheme of a full life. Really, it's a blip on the radar. There is so much to look forward to, so much to anticipate together in the years ahead. A period of sexual longing or urgency might even do a couple good and can set them up for some long-lasting passion.

Keep all of this in mind when you are on your way to the hospital, or when you are sitting next to your wife in that chemo room. The best is yet to come. Even in bed. Or on the kitchen floor. Whatever you prefer! Just make sure the kids are at Grandma's house.

ဢ႗ၺ

First Person

I was working when my wife received the mammography report that revealed she had breast cancer. Between this mammography result and the biopsy, however, it seemed like everything was in slow motion. All of the reports and the initial doctor's appointments seemed very slow, I suppose because we were anxious to begin making decisions. We were on the edge of our chairs.

I did accompany my wife to all of the doctors' appointments, but I purposefully withheld my thoughts and opinions about what she should do. A big part of her consideration was whether to have a single mastectomy or a double. I knew that it would ultimately be her decision because it is her body.

Although we had a lot of appointments with surgeons and therapists, the surgery itself seemed to arrive quickly. I wasn't too worried about the surgery, I was primarily just concerned that they would be able to get at all of the cancer.

The hardest part was the chemotherapy afterward. This lasted about three to four months. It primarily made my wife very tired. I would leave her at home in the morning, go to work, and return to find her in much the same position as when I left. I knew she was just worn out. But I know that chemo affects all women differently. During the chemo, I would say that her conversations were muted, she was slow in speech and response, and she might have been feeling depressed. This was difficult for her. It was like she was living under an overcast sky constantly.

But she made it through this first bout, and we were able to make several life changes, including my retirement.

Some years later, cancer was discovered in the lymph nodes, and she had to return for a second surgery and therapy. I don't know how to compare the two experiences—they were both so different, and it was at a different time in our lives.

After this second surgery to remove the cancer, she had another round of chemotherapy, which was different than the first, and this was followed by radiation, which affected her in other ways. As opposed to the washed-out feeling that chemotherapy gave her, now she had to struggle with radiation scarring and a raw throat. I believe I had to take her to the emergency room once because she could not swallow and the pain was too intense.

Naturally, I'd recommend that no one have to go through this. Cancer is not for the faint of heart.

~Bob

ဆၢ

My wife is a very independent and take-charge woman, and the first time I heard about my wife's breast cancer was when she told me. But she had already made decisions about what she was doing to do and what would be required. She had talked to the doctors, done her research, and made all of the decisions before I even knew about the cancer.

I knew both of us would do whatever was required through surgery and treatment. Whether it was housework or transportation, it was not a problem for me; I just knew what I had to do and did it.

My wife has always had that spirit: "Here is the challenge, and here is what we are going to do about it."

But breast cancer impacted us in other ways. Cancer really makes a person think about mortality, and cancer changed the way we think about prayer and worship. We had a lot of time during all of the radiation and chemo to think about these things. And although it was difficult for me to watch so many people taking the chemo treatments, I made a point of staying upbeat. It would be easy to get depressed.

In many ways cancer made us both more positive people and gave us a stronger marriage. I think women fear losing their breasts like men fear losing their manhood, but to me nothing changed about my wife. She has always been the same person.

~Anonymous

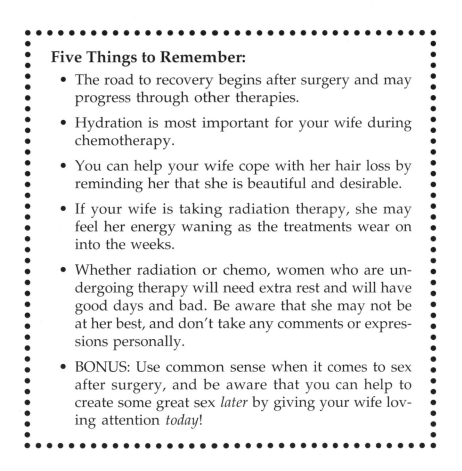

Five Things to Remember:

- The road to recovery begins after surgery and may progress through other therapies.

- Hydration is most important for your wife during chemotherapy.

- You can help your wife cope with her hair loss by reminding her that she is beautiful and desirable.

- If your wife is taking radiation therapy, she may feel her energy waning as the treatments wear on into the weeks.

- Whether radiation or chemo, women who are undergoing therapy will need extra rest and will have good days and bad. Be aware that she may not be at her best, and don't take any comments or expressions personally.

- BONUS: Use common sense when it comes to sex after surgery, and be aware that you can help to create some great sex *later* by giving your wife loving attention *today*!

Husband's Quick Guide to Breast Cancer Recovery

Top 10 Things to Remember

1. The longer you live past the breast cancer diagnosis, the less you will think of your wife as a breast cancer survivor.

2. As the years go by, your wife's scars will fade and life will return to "normal".

3. After you have lived through the worst of the treatments, plan to go away together on a celebratory trip.

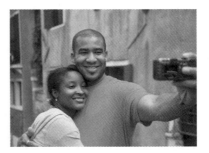

4. Re-energize your lives by making changes to your diet.

5. Plan to exercise together.

6. Pursue your individual hobbies, but find something you can also enjoy together.

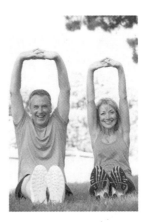

7. Remember your wife's breast cancer diagnosis (date) every year by acknowledging your love for her.

8. Encourage your wife to help other women who have been diagnosed if she feels like getting involved.

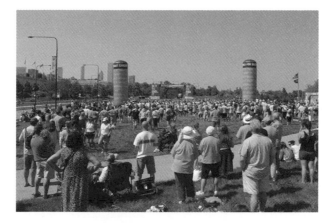

9. If your wife does get involved, participate in some events with her.

10. Allow your life to return to a new "normal," but don't be surprised if you also live differently following breast cancer.

Chapter Eight
Facing the Future After Breast Cancer

Eventually every breast cancer survivor—every family—desires to get back to "normal." But in many respects, the old life is difficult to recover. In fact, there will be much in your life that will not be the same.

Don't forget: your wife has certainly been changed through this experience. She may feel she has been given a second chance at life, or she may have a heightened sense of her purpose or her goals. She may have a keener sense of her own mortality. You may, indeed, experience a woman who loves and feels more deeply than ever before. Perhaps she is more spiritual or more in touch the people around her. Or she may grow more introspective and quiet as the months pass, and you will wonder what she is thinking.

In truth, there is no "normal" for breast cancer survivors.

Nevertheless, there are certain experiences and periods that most breast cancer survivors and families journey through, so let's talk about them.

The First Two Years

For the two years following surgery and treatment, most women will harbor some lingering fears about the recurrence of breast cancer or discovery of cancer elsewhere. This may be more "normal" or natural than not thinking about cancer at all. The signs of breast cancer will also be evident during this period.

When a woman looks in the mirror, she may still see evidence of a lumpectomy, a dent in her breast where a portion of tissue was removed. Or she may see her mastectomy scar every morning when she gets out of the shower or have a sensory awareness of her breast implant. Likewise, she may still be thinking about her prosthesis, or have a wig or two lying around (post-chemo), or see no breast at all. She may also be more aware of how her scars or chemotherapy still linger in her body, but how the memory, like the changing color of the scar itself, is fading over time. She is

131

getting back to "normal", but is not quite there yet. There is still a freshness to the cancer experience, and you might even note from time to time how much the scar is fading or how she is returning to her old self.

All of these experiences can be a part of these early years, and there is no one way that women live them. The mirror is still in play during these early months, and women will often note how their bodies continue to change and adapt; some may begin to feel certain twinges of sorrow or, from time to time, be overcome with emotion.

Men can be especially helpful during this early period by reminding their wives they look beautiful and by encouraging them through their periodic bouts with fear. If a woman needs affirmation, provide it.

During this time, women will also have a couple of checkups (mammograms, etc.). These can be particularly scary, so be sure you mark these dates on your calendar, too, and make it a special point to do something together on these days. These appointment dates will be crucial to note, because many women experience bouts of depression at these junctures. Being reminded, once again, of the realities of losing a breast or of having to have the body checked for cancer can be a depressing day. Consider these anniversaries if you discover that your wife is edgy or morose when the dates roll around.

Women who have undergone radiation or chemo will also have a unique set of feelings during this initial stage. These therapies consume a great deal of energy and emotion, and in many respects the therapies establish disciplines and bonds that then have their own set of loss attached to them when they are no longer there. Many women feel a sense of security through the chemo experience, and when it finally comes to an end, there can be a sense of depression. Other women feel they should continue the treatments. It's like losing a trusted ally, a dependable friend.

One of our dear friends experienced this type of disconnection following the end of her chemotherapy. She felt at loose ends for some weeks, even too free, as her weeks had been regimented so closely by the high and low tides of the chemo. Without it, she had to relearn everything from exercise to diet. Being free of the chemo was actually the first step in her cancer-free life, and for a time she was at loose ends.

Make this a special time for your wife. If she is undergoing chemo or radiation, be sure to at least acknowledge the milestone, and if possible, have a celebration. Invite friends in for dinner. Have a family gathering. Throw a party. Do something to acknowledge that this is a new beginning, and your wife will appreciate the encouragement, too.

The first two years after surgery can also be a time of adjustment for the two of you. Perhaps you have found yourselves talking about breast cancer too much (after all, there is more to your lives than breast cancer, and no one should talk themselves to death about it). Perhaps your conversations are too centered on these thoughts, and you need to find more uplifting topics. You may also be working on new ventures together or setting new goals. These are vital. This adjustment period may also include life changes or changes in family needs that have followed on the heels of the breast cancer. You may have discovered a new joy in your children, for example, or taken on a new career path.

Finally, you may discover that you are still finding each other during this initial period. Some couples I know have described this period much in the same terms as a "second honeymoon." Post-surgery couples may have to work at discovering their sexual chemistry or sexual intimacy again.

During these two years, it will be important to keep an open but active mind and to be aware of what your wife is feeling. You are making these adjustments together.

After Five Years

Five years is another milestone in the breast cancer experience. After five years, most breast cancer survivors have discovered a cadence to their lives. Bouts of mild depression are generally not as pronounced, and most women do not think about breast cancer as often. In fact, you are probably not aware of how little you do think about a missing breast or the aftermath of chemo. A kind of normalcy returns to the family.

The five-year mark is a milestone for many women, as breast cancer then begins to feel more like a distant memory, as some vestige of a former life. By now the harsh appearance of scarring has faded, the aftermath of chemo (such as hair regrowth and certain other side effects) is no longer an issue, and most couples have settled into routines that have little or nothing to do with the breast cancer journey.

My wife has always advocated that the five-year mark is an important one for breast cancer survivors. She says that, up until that point, she thought about cancer frequently, worried about checkups, and was aware of her survivor status every time she looked in the mirror. But as time passed, there developed a kind of normalcy to the experience.

Five years is important.

At this juncture, however, many women may notice their energies are not the same as they once were. Perhaps the toll of career and family has once again settled upon them, and they are engaged in many activities. This is not all-together a bad thing; it demonstrates that breast cancer no longer defines their lives.

Many women also begin to think about how they can support others in their journeys with cancer. Some women will become active in support groups, or sign up for a Susan B. Komen walk, for example. More women may discover they are able to talk about their experiences with other women who have been recently diagnosed. In short, after five years or so, most women are more reflective about their experiences and can talk about cancer without the raw emotion.

Men can note this milestone and continue to be supportive by encouraging their wives to participate in cancer walks, support groups or charity events. I know that my wife spent dozens of hours on the telephone counseling other women around this time, and I was proud she was able to be so helpful and articulate.

The five-year mark can be a key celebration in many ways.

Beyond Seven Years

After seven years, breast cancer survivors enter yet another phase. Now, cancer is no longer on her mind as it once was, and should there be a recurrence of cancer, doctors would regard it as a new manifestation not connected with the original diagnosis and treatment.

There can be other important milestones, too.

In fact, during the writing of this paragraph, I note that my wife completed the final leg of her clinical trial/study the night before. I had accompanied her to her final MRI diagnostic (eleven years past treatment) on her breast implant. She felt relieved to complete this leg of the journey and was looking forward to receiving her last small stipend from participating in the trial—a stipend she would use to reward herself with a new piece of motorcycle-riding attire. We had dinner together following the MRI to celebrate her release from the study and wondered what the trials would reveal. Beyond this, breast cancer is not something we readily think about anymore or even acknowledge—certainly not on a daily basis.

So, even at ten years and beyond, there are milestones that can be celebrated. The disease no longer has the same influence and power it once had. It's something of a distant memory. So much has happened, and after seven years most women no longer feel the emotional punch of the "C" word.

In the event your wife is still coping with cancer after seven years (because of a recurrence or participation in a study), it might be helpful to read further in chapter ten (When You Need Help). This is to acknowledge that not all women are cancer-free after ten years. Some families are still touched by breast cancer in a big way, and so seven years and beyond may have a different feel to these couples. Seven years may not feel like the end, but rather the beginning.

ᔕᘓᘎ

First Person

I can't say that, after fifteen years, my wife and I even think about breast cancer very much. We don't think about it in the same way, certainly. We do worry about our daughter, sometimes, and wonder if these things could be hereditary. But breast cancer has in one way defined our future or dictated how we have lived since.

Yes, I'd say that there were milestones along the way. We've moved, built a new house, and had our celebrations. But as time has passed, the cancer experience seems disconnected from where we've been.

I remember once, reading about _____(a famous writer) whose wife was diagnosed with breast cancer. His wife was worried that he wouldn't find her attractive after her mastectomy or that he would leave her for a larger-breasted woman. He just made jokes about it, and this added some comic relief that seemed to help.

I think humor has helped us, too. You know, life's too short to worry through it. Like we've learned from many other roads, there are many things in life we can't change; we just have to deal with them. I think this is true for breast cancer, too.

Sure, I've changed along the way—mainly gotten older and grayer—but with each passing year I'm just grateful we've had our health. Breast cancer is rough, but for most women like my wife, it's not the end of life. That's not true for everyone. So we feel fortunate.

Make every day count. That's what I've learned. Live and enjoy each other. You use fewer face muscles when you smile. I read that somewhere. I think it's true. That's really helped us. I'd recommend it.

~Frank

Five Things to Remember:

- The stages after cancer treatment are important.

- Depression is more common early on and during anniversaries (such as the diagnosis date, surgery date, etc.).

- Men can help by remembering milestones and by celebrating the end of therapy with their wives.

- As time passes, women will be able to express their thoughts about the cancer experience and begin helping others.

- Be thankful for each day.

Chapter Nine
Learning to Help Yourself

Many men will tell you that it is difficult to be the caregiver and have a life at the same time. Many men feel like they have given up a life to help their wives, and some grow to resent it. You don't want that to happen.

Recently I was talking to a group of men who were part of a grief-recovery workshop, and a couple of them were honest enough to express these thoughts:

- "Men usually suffer silently, and even if they could talk about their anger or resentment, they probably don't."

- "I didn't realize how much time I was spending at home until after the football season. I hadn't watched a single game, and no one had invited me over for a Super Bowl party. I guess all my friends assumed I couldn't attend. But it was lonely."

- "I think that by concentrating on my wife's needs for so long, I was actually denying my own feelings—especially anger—and I had to come to terms with myself again."

- "It was amazing how much of myself I lost in this process of breast cancer. The first time I had an evening to myself I felt like a kid again."

It is not easy to express feelings such as these. Sometimes men don't want to look this deep into their own pain or grief. For some, it might be the most difficult thing they will ever do.

Being the caregiver through the breast cancer journey is not for the faint-hearted. It does take stamina and dedication. It takes love and self-sacrifice.

In another session, one man handed me an article he had clipped from a magazine. The headline read, *"The Silent Cry of the Caregiver."* Aptly named, this piece described how most men suffer in silence, but inside they are screaming to express what they want and need. This is especially true when we are helping a wife through a serious illness such as breast cancer.

If you are feeling like you need to rediscover yourself or find your life or your pace again, here are some simple guidelines that might help. Nothing earth-shattering here, but at least you will know that your internal struggles are recognized. That in itself is often the best medicine.

Voice Recognition—Finding Yourself Again

Sooner or later you will need to reestablish some of your old patterns, which may be the disciplines that have served you well in your life up to this point. One of the reasons we all have daily routines is because they save us time and energy and allow us to concentrate our mental energies on more important and creative matters. The routines—such as brushing our teeth, showering and shaving, combing our hair, and driving the same route to work—don't expend much mental energy, but they do allow us to dream and create while we are doing them. (I don't think dentists get this, however; it's why we don't concentrate our mental energy on brushing and flossing the proper way!)

Once your caregiving days are over, you need to get back to some of these old ways. It may be that you have fallen out of morning routines, or perhaps you have been hurrying home (instead of stopping in at the gym or the softball field). Well, now you are free to return to these pursuits. By doing them, slowly you will feel like you are reclaiming your life. You'll actually feel more energized, less anxious and angry, and will probably sleep more soundly.

You may also have fallen away from your diet. I know many men who, during their caregiving days, either gain a good deal of weight or lose too much too quickly. Stress can do that to us. It will be important for you to reestablish these good diet patterns. I'm not saying that if you are accustomed to a steady diet of fast food, you should return to it. No! Rather, you simply need to get back to what you enjoy. Eat well, of course, but don't forget to take care of yourself.

Sometimes men neglect friendships. After showering your wife with so much attention, it may be time to shower your friends with some, also. They have probably missed you, and while many of them may have been there for you, others may have dropped off the map. It might be time to reestablish some of these friendships with a phone call or a golf outing. And if there are certain friends who went above and beyond the call in their helpfulness, how about buying a round of beers?

Perhaps your hobbies have suffered, as well. I've known some men who have sold motorcycles, swapped cars, or even cashed in their golf clubs in order to attend to their wife's needs. Admirable, yes. But some of these decisions left nothing in the bank. Now and again a guy has to redeem some of his own stock in order to keep himself strong. So don't neglect returning to that rock-climbing or your favorite bowling alley.

And while we're on the subject, let's talk about sex. A lot of men express angst over the changing patterns of their sex lives during and soon after the breast cancer experience. It is true that your wife may not have felt amorous after her surgery or during chemo. And if your sex life hasn't returned to its previous robust levels, don't pout about it. Make plans.

Chances are your wife may be feeling a little neglected or cheated, as well. The recovery period is a great time to actually discuss your sex life and heat things up. As noted earlier, breast cancer has a way of changing women's feelings about sex, too, and often they emerge from their treatment and recovery period with a newfound eagerness in the sack. If your sex life has grown a bit lackluster over the months, don't assume that's the way it is going to be future tense. Make some plans together and begin to talk about your sex life. Things might heat up faster than you realize, and some men report that the sex they enjoy post-cancer is more intense than before. This might have more to do with *her* than with *you*! But don't debate the reasons. Just do it.

Finally, you can reclaim your life by taking on some new pursuits. You have probably learned a great deal about yourself, and maybe you even see life differently now, because of the breast cancer journey. Dream a dream. Make it a point to try something daring. One guy I know, during his wife's breast cancer struggle,

141

actually took to skydiving. I'm not suggesting you jump from 20,000 feet, but there is probably a pursuit you've always wanted to try. Whether it be painting or hiking or riding a motorcycle—find that one new thing that can make you feel you've got your life back. You'll thank yourself for this many times in the years ahead.

෯෬

First Person

I was really slow to make changes after caring for my wife for six months. It wasn't around-the-clock care, but it was intense enough for me. I went with her to every doctor's appointment and chemo treatment. She lost her appetite for a while and I had to order certain foods. I'm not saying I resented any of this; I would do it again in a heartbeat. But I did put a lot of my pursuits to the side. Most of them I didn't miss at all. But there was work I didn't get done and at least one promotion I may have missed because of it. Oh, well.

What I did do later, after my wife was well, was learn how to play the guitar. It's something I have always wanted to do. I thought I could reward myself that way. I'm glad I did. I enjoy playing, and some day I hope I can be good enough to get up a garage band. Who knows?

I didn't want to be selfish during my wife's illness. I guess I devoted most of my energy toward her. It's all good. She's fine now. Thank God.

But what I do think is important is reinventing yourself after it is all over. Not big changes, mind you—I don't think more change is what I needed. I just wanted to take on some new adventure for myself, and it was very therapeutic. I think every man should do it.

~Mike

Five Things to Remember

- You need to reestablish routines in order to regain your creative mind.

- Reestablish your friendships.

- Pursue your hobbies.

- Re-create and refresh your sex life.

- Do something new for yourself.

Chapter Ten
When You Need Help

During the months I was interviewing men and writing this book, one question continued to emerge: "What if?" The question was posed in a variety of ways. *"What if* my wife is diagnosed with an advanced stage of cancer?" *"What if* the cancer returns?" *"What if* the surgery and treatment had not been effective?"

There were a few men who wondered, "What if the cancer could not be treated?" or "What if my wife died?"

The fact is, while breast cancer is certainly not a death sentence to most women, it is nevertheless a serious disease. Some women do have protracted battles. Some women die.

If you find yourself asking one of those "what if" questions, read on. Some of your questions may be addressed in the pages ahead, though perhaps not answered. Nevertheless, no man should have to journey through his caregiving alone, and there are valuable insights and resources that can help you if you are caring for a wife who has been diagnosed with an advanced, or in some cases terminal, form of cancer.

In recent years there have been a number of memoirs written from a woman's perspective about caring for a husband with a terminal cancer condition (Joan Didion's *The Year of Magical Thinking* and Joyce Carol Oates's *A Widow's Story* are two among a myriad of others). However, it is rare to find a memoir written from a man's perspective.

There is much we can learn from other men who have walked the walk, and if we pad about in their shoes for a while and listen to their stories, they can teach us how to do long-term care, or how to care at the end of life. Their testimonies are memoirs. And it is helpful to hear the stories of men who drive to work each day and still find time to do the difficult work of caring for a sick wife.

Not every man, of course, does well in this role. Many men, whether they would admit it or not, struggle. We like to fix things.

And when we can't fix it, we often grow frustrated or despondent. And metastatic cancer is not a battle we can fix on our own.

Each year, less than five percent of all women diagnosed with breast cancer end up battling a metastatic pathology. Most breast cancers are confined to the breasts or surrounding tissues and can be treated through surgery, radiation or chemo to the pectoral region. However, in this small portion of women, metastatic forms of cancer do develop. Sometimes the cancer is not detected until a more advanced stage, when it has already spread to other organs. Or sometimes the tumor is large, and the margins for removing it are difficult to obtain. And sometimes there are certain forms of cancer that simply spread quickly. Age also plays a factor. Younger women often have more aggressive forms of cancer, as the body is still producing healthy cells, and the cancer can spread more rapidly to other parts of the body. And as noted before, family history and genetic predisposition to cancer can also play a large role in the type of cancer and its metastatic manifestations. Scientists are still uncertain about all of these factors, and discoveries linked to our DNA and genetic makeup are being made, it seems, every year.

But until a cure for cancer is found, we know that a certain percentage of women will battle metastatic cancer. And some of this cancer will have originated in the breast(s).

When a loved one, however, is battling against cancer or fighting against time, we don't really care about statistics and interesting facts or potential cures. We simply want to help our loved ones through their crisis. We may not need answers, but we do need help.

And that's where a husband can make all the difference in the world.

Being the Lifeline

In the event that your wife has an ongoing battle on her hands—perhaps facing additional chemotherapy, surgeries, or even experimental treatments—there is much you should know. There is much to do. And everything you do will have great significance to your wife.

In many respects, you will become the lifeline. You will be more than just a caregiver; you will be the care itself.

In the event you have a more protracted battle plan, here are more than a dozen important things to remember:

Bad Days

Be aware that your wife may have many more "bad" days than "good" ones, meaning that she may grow increasingly weak or have much longer or protracted bouts with weakness, nausea, fatigue or restlessness. She may simply want to sleep, or she may draw into herself more frequently (or meditate or pray) in order to find the internal peace she is seeking. Keep in mind, these bad days are not a reflection on you; it's just that your wife may not feel well enough to engage in long conversations, or entertainment, or even her usual pursuits. Sometimes women who are deep in the throes of chemo will simply be worn out. They may not have enough energy for others, as her energy must be internalized to fight the disease. So don't let "bad" days get *you* down! Give your wife her space on these days; allow her to rest, sleep or rejuvenate. Hopefully the bad day will be followed by a good day, or a string of them. You can help your wife recover faster by honoring the bad times.

Appetite and Food

Chemo and radiation therapy can impact not only a patient's appetite, but also the appeal of food in general, or even the type of food. Some cancer patients, for example, may find certain foods or aromas repulsive. Favorite foods and tastes can often change on the tongue during therapy, and so nothing can be taken for granted in terms of "the usual" fare. Be prepared to deal with your wife's appetite changes. Be prepared to experiment with new food or with "what sounds good" to her in the moment. Some women may go through periods when only certain flavors of gelatin, certain soups, or even dry, unsalted crackers are the only fare that appeals.

Other women don't seem to be impacted by the chemo in this way and may stay on their diets throughout the treatments. There's no telling. Some men have noted that chemo and radiation can have a marked resemblance to pregnancy, with their wives craving certain foods at strange hours of the day, or losing an appetite, only to rediscover an insatiable hunger a few hours later. Be prepared for anything. And again, don't lose heart in your own cooking skills or think that you have failed if you can't meet the need. Ask for help. You may have a friend, neighbor or other family member who could even step in for a time and cook your wife's favorites.

Other men I have known have asked their wives to prepare menus beforehand, along with step-by-step recipes, so they can cook without making mistakes. Their wives feel they are participating in their own care but also receiving care at the same time. And then, of course, there are those men who may cook better than their wives, anyway. You might be one. Lucky for you.

Respect Her Needs

Some men note that their wives can become more demanding during their illness or as the breast cancer struggle wears on. But this should be expected. Some of these demands may come about as a need for security or even comfort. So respect what she needs (and even what she is requesting).

Some women may need help you cannot provide, such as help while you are working, or assistance in the middle of the night or in preparing certain foods. That's when you will need to reach out to others and ask for help.

One family I know took turns helping out in the house, with sisters, children, parents and husband all taking turns around the clock to give constant care to their loved one. That way, no single caregiver was responsible for all of the care, and no one got worn out or angry. Through shared responsibilities, this family truly knew the meaning of caregiving and turned it into "care-living."

Be sure to ask your wife what she needs and make a list of these things as you go through the journey with her. Be attentive to her needs first, and everything else will fall into place.

Give Her Space

Even though she may be weak or struggling, it is important to give your wife some personal space. This space is important for several reasons.

First, be aware that the noise factor in a house can be heightened for a person who is ill from chemo or low on energy. A loud TV, a blaring radio, or even boisterous family laughter can seem like nails raking across a chalkboard. Never assume that what you are hearing is what she is hearing. You may be hearing soothing music. To her, the music could be grating and shrill. Every day, make it a point to ask about her comfort and her space. Is she comfortable?

Secondly, what she sees is also important. Remember, she may not be able to move about and manage her own sight lines as easily as you. Are family photos comforting? Are they worrisome? Is the TV on? Would she prefer not to have the TV on? Is the sun too bright? Would she prefer the shades open? You see where this is going. Make sure her space is comfortable, and never assume that what you see is what she sees from her vantage point. Be vigilant.

Finally, and this may be most important, actually respect her space. There may be times when your wife will simply want to *be*. Everyone needs a space like this. And since she may not be able to find that space on her own (because she is too weak, too sick, or has no motivation, etc.), you may need to help her by providing it. Let her enjoy where she is, and if she wants to be alone for a while, respect her privacy and her need for peace and quiet. Step away, or ask her when you should check back. Her space is important, and if there are items she would like in her area, bring them. It's all good, and by giving her space you will also be allowing yourself (and giving yourself) permission to rest a bit. Everyone needs quiet in order to refuel. And if your wife is fighting a hard battle, give her a respite so she can draw inside herself and get stronger.

Help Her With Meds

Many women eventually reach a point where they need help regulating or keeping track of their medications. Those pill sorters (by day or week) are a helpful tool, and men don't have to feel like a nurse in order to be effective. Take a look at all labels, make a record of when each medication should be taken, create a day-by-day or hour-by-hour outline, and then go do it.

The medication help is especially needed when it comes to pain management. If you don't have professional help and must manage some of this on your own, be especially vigilant.

Buffer Visitors

This can also include phone calls and emails—even letters. Be certain your wife is not overwhelmed with people or information.

Men can be most helpful to their wives by buffering visitors at certain times. For example, you may know your wife's "good days" and "bad days" based on the chemo or radiation schedule. In time, a pattern develops, and you get a clear picture of the days and hours and how your wife is responding to the therapy.

By buffering visitors (or phone calls, etc.) on the bad days, you can help your wife immensely. This doesn't mean you are rude to your family and friends, but believe me, everyone understands if you simply say, "My wife isn't feeling her best today, but she would like to see you (talk to you) another time. Thanks so much for thinking of her and for your concern."

Buffering visitors can hearken back to giving your wife space for recovery, and it can also provide a more consistent flow through the breast cancer journey. As anyone who has ever had a lengthy stay in a hospital can attest, the hospital is no place to rest. There are always interruptions, conversations, tests, probes and jabs. A constant stream of visitors doesn't always help us when we are ill. You can help provide this consistency.

One final note on visitors. As a pastor, I have called on thousands of people during times of illness. If you do have a pastor or religious leader, don't hesitate to suggest times and dates that would be optimal for a visit. In fact, they would appreciate the guidance.

Finally, if you do have a lot of other correspondence that is getting backlogged (letters, cards, emails from family and friends), ask your wife about the best time to give these to her, or even read them to her. She probably would enjoy these expressions of care as much or more than a lengthy visit, anyway. These can also be special times for the two of you, when you can open these and read them together.

Be Her Smile

Your wife married you for many reasons. One of those reasons had to be your smile—your humor, the joy you bring to her life.

When your wife is battling cancer, don't forget to be her sunshine. This may sound hokey, or even overly sentimental or maudlin, but if you are dour, she is going to feel it. Find your best face, in fact always put on your best face, when you speak to her. Regardless of what has happened in your world (at work, with the family, or what is going on in the universe), be present with your wife in a positive way. Your wife, in fact, needs your smile and your positive outlook just as much as she needs her treatments. Never underestimate your role in your wife's healing or her journey through cancer.

One fellow I knew years back told me he helped his wife through cancer in a very unusual way. Every night, before they went to bed, they told jokes. Sometimes he bought joke books, or wrote silly limericks, or read from volumes of humorous stories. But he claims the laughter was truly the best medicine.

So don't overlook the gift of your smile when it comes to making your wife's day.

Pamper Her

Your wife deserves to be pampered, and there are many ways you can soothe her and help her to relax. Some of these might include giving her a back rub, a foot rub, or actually bringing in a massage therapist who specializes in this type of care. Your wife might also enjoy having special scrapbooks of family history or photographs prepared for her or, perhaps, watching a favorite movie some evening.

If your wife still has an appetite, you might also consider making some of her favorite meals. A gift basket can be a nice gesture, too, and even items such as hand lotions and body lotions can be a soothing comfort to a tired body. These small gifts can make her feel very special.

Allow Her to Vent

There may be days where your wife simply needs to cry or express bitterness, resentment or even anger. Remember, most of us only express such feelings with those we feel closest to. Honesty comes when we feel a level of comfort, of vulnerability.

Give your wife permission to vent. Tell her you will listen to anything she wants to say, even if it is harsh, abrasive or brutally honest. You may be the only person she can speak to, the only one who will listen to her frustrations. She might even express herself with a depth you have never seen before. But when a woman can do this, she can feel unburdened, fresh, and new. Many men may feel very uncomfortable in these situations, but if you just listen and don't try to offer solutions or fix the problem, it is enough. Just let her know she has been heard. You care. You are listening.

Provide Consistency

Nothing can be more debilitating than boredom. You can help alleviate this by providing consistency to your wife's day, especially by making sure she can continue some of her favorite activities and hobbies, even if she is too weak to move about. For example, your wife might enjoy doing the morning crossword puzzle in the newspaper (and you can help). Or she might enjoy knitting or crochet work. Be aware of the items she might need, even if she can only work at them for minutes at a time.

Your wife might also like some playing cards for solitaire, or perhaps some sudoku books, word searches, or word games. She might like to read but might also need a better reading lamp, some more powerful reading glasses, or even a magnifying glass. Keep her well-stocked with her favorite hobbies.

You don't have to be overbearing in this department, just make sure she doesn't slip into boredom or feel lonely and worried. Worry is alleviated, in part, when our minds are occupied elsewhere, especially on fun or rewarding pursuits. You have fun, too. Do something together. You'll both enjoy it.

Make Her Comfortable

There are many ways you can make your wife more comfortable. Be sure to ask. She may prefer soft, soothing music. Aromatherapy is pleasurable for many women, or sometimes just burning a scented candle can be relaxing. New silk or flannel sheets and some softer pillows can add comfort. A bathrobe might be very appealing to her, or even some pajamas.

Lift Her Spirits

During times of crisis, most people will draw strength from their faith or spirituality. For some people this strength may be found through their faith tradition or through spiritual practices they have developed (such as prayer, meditation, study or silence). Even if you and your wife don't practice a faith or have any particular beliefs, that doesn't mean your wife doesn't have a need to strengthen her spirit, or her resolve. You can help lift her spirits, too.

If your wife does have a faith, be sure to encourage her to pray or study or participate in those disciplines that are meaningful to her—that can help her to connect to God. You could also buy her books, CDs, DVDs or other inspirational material. Your place of worship might also have recommendations.

If you and your wife are accustomed to praying together, you should certainly continue this practice. Seeking God together is important, and if you are able to share these special moments spiritually, you should not shy away from them.

End-of-Life Issues

As a pastor I am intimately acquainted with the end of life. I have the privilege (and it is a privilege afforded to few) of being present to people while they are taking their final breath. I have been blessed by families who have allowed me to hold their hands, to be present with their loved ones, to say final words, to offer comfort and meaning. Death is never easy. But there are certainly many disciplines that can help us cope with life's final passage and also make it easier for us to help a loved one die. Some of these issues belong to the living. But other factors are made easier, or more difficult, because of the spirit and acceptance of the individual who is dying.

So, let me offer a few insights here that can help those husbands whose wives have terminal cancer.

As is noted in Elizabeth Kubler-Ross's classic volume *On Death and Dying*, terminal patients go through several emotional stages prior to death. These various stages are not experienced in any particular order, nor even by every patient, but most individuals do go through periods of questioning, denial and despair before arriving at a place of acceptance. There can be other stages, as well, but for women who are dying of breast cancer, there can also be disbelief and withdrawal. No husband can go wrong with reading Kubler-Ross's work; the book has sold millions of copies in no small part because her insights are so universally accurate and applicable for cancer patients.

Husbands will also go through many of these same stages, but in a different fashion. Instead of experiencing a physical death, a husband may experience grief associated with the loss of a love, of a relationship, of one's hopes and dreams. Many men, at first, will deny the reality of death, or hold out the hope that a miracle cure will be forthcoming, or even ignore the inevitable. But sooner or later these same men will come to accept their role as a caregiver at the end of life. These stages are never easy, and death is always fraught with an enormous emotional toll. Kubler-Ross's book *On Grief and Grieving* is another classic that speaks to these concerns. Men who are faced with providing care for their wives will do well to read this work for their own peace of mind.

During over thirty years of pastoral ministry, I have witnessed many men who have risen to the occasion and provided this final care for their wives. These men have always amazed me, and some have noted to me later that those final days with their wives were filled with some of the most remarkable conversations and insights about life.

There are many examples I could give, stories I could tell, but suffice it to say that men have an uncanny ability to exhibit strength in the midst of adversity. Perhaps we are built that way, but we are at our best, it seems, when the chips are down. So don't doubt that you have the resiliency and fortitude to make your wife's final weeks both comfortable and remarkable.

For those who desire a more accessible and practical approach to helping their wives at the end of life, let me offer here some insights gleaned from my years of ministry and from watching other men's experience.

- At some point your wife will want to talk about her death. Don't dismiss this or ignore her words. This is part of the grieving and acceptance process and is vital to her ability to cope well with her death. No one is helped if we do not speak of death, or if we pretend it does not exist or cannot touch us. It is okay—in fact, it is healthy—to use the word "death" instead of catch phrases like "passing away" or "crossing over" or "making the journey." When your wife is ready to talk about her death, she will let you know. This may be a few weeks before, or days before, or in some cases just hours prior to death—but when that time comes, be prepared to listen and offer your own acceptance and love. There is no way I can tell you what to say, but you can't go wrong with expressing your love, affirming you will miss her, and detailing how much she has meant to you and the family.

- There are many ways we can face death nobly and meaningfully. Some of these may involve a faith tradition or certain beliefs about the life to come. Don't hesitate to offer this hope together and speak of it, and if you need help, don't hesitate to call your priest or pastor, for example.

- If your wife has any final plans or requests, be sure to listen for these. A woman may not always articulate these specifically, but if you listen closely, you can probably ascertain what some of her final wishes might be.

- Whether early in the dying process or later, you will likely want to contact hospice care. Hospice will see that your wife is comfortable and pain-free, and they

155

will help the entire family through the grieving and dying process. Hospice does this very well, and I have encountered very few people who have not had wonderful experiences with hospice.

- If you have a will, be sure to review it. Be sure that your wife works on her Last Will and Testament before she becomes too ill. Don't put these tasks off due to denial or an inability to discuss the implications of death. Be prepared.

- Your wife may want to express some wishes or ideas about her funeral service or memorial. Again, don't downplay this or ignore her desire to talk about it. Accept that this is a healthy step, and allow your wife to discuss these matters with you.

- Remember , discussing these matters may be more difficult for you than it is for her. But just because these matters make you feel uncomfortable, don't deny their importance for your wife's mental health. Allow her to talk about these matters when she is ready. Then step in and listen.

- Acknowledge your wife's feelings. Again, this is vital, as you don't want to pretend your wife is not in pain, or deny she is uncomfortable, or pretend she has an appetite. If your wife tells you she is not hungry or she doesn't feel like eating, don't try to force her to eat a meal. She will only grow to resent your efforts and will assume you are out of touch with her situation. Let her be the guide.

- If pain management is needed, make sure you have the phone numbers handy of your visiting nurses or hospice workers. They will usually be present or be able to give you guidance.

- Be near your wife. You don't just want to be inside the same four walls. You want to be by her side.

There is no way that all matters related to death and dying can be related in a brief summary such as this. But rest assured that you can't go wrong with being available and caring. Anything you wish to express to your wife should be on the table, too. You may find that, while your heart is breaking, it is also filled with gratitude. Tell your wife how much you appreciate her, why she is special to you, why you love her, and be sure to share special memories. Relive some of your favorite places and moments in life. This may seem sad at the outset, but most men find this exercise surprisingly fulfilling and comforting.

A great many cancer-related books don't deal with end-of-life issues, but for those men who need this help, the information is crucial. There are also many Web sites and resources available for men—help that can add much more to the conversation and make these end-of-life issues more tolerable.

Check out the various Web sites at the back of this book. I'm sure you can find one or two there that deal specifically in caregiving at the end of life or serve as catalysts to help men discuss these issues in a safe and discrete forum.

₧₧₧

First Person

We found out my wife had a lump in the breast in early November, and two months later, in January, she had a mastectomy followed by chemo and radiation. We knew at the time that she had a Stage 4 cancer, but my wife and our family, along with the doctors, thought that she had beaten it.

Four-and-a-half years later she returned from her annual checkup with the news that the cancer had returned and was in a lung. Naturally, she began to second guess her previous decisions. She wondered how her prognosis would have been different if she had had both breasts removed, or if she had taken additional treatments.

When we returned to the doctor to begin treatment for this metastatic cancer in the lung, he was not very positive with me and the family, and yet he told us that we had to remain positive and not let my wife lose hope. This was very difficult, but I took that as my personal responsibility and was how I approached every day. What also made this difficult for me was that I wanted to make the cancer go away, I wanted to make things different for my wife, but I could not. I felt like I was unable to make her comfortable, either physically or emotionally. She did go through periods of extreme pain and eight different chemo drugs.

This second journey with the cancer was quite different from the first. As my wife began taking a harsher form of chemo, she developed the "chemo brain" that people talk about. She was not always logical, and often her needs were confused and confusing to the family. We had a family gathering at our house, for example, and in the middle of our time together my wife grew very bitter and asked everyone to leave the house: children, grandchildren, everyone. This was very difficult, but we didn't want to upset her any further, so the day was over.

As my wife grew nearer to the end of life, she needed more medication, and so I was accelerating the frequency and trying to meet her needs that way. I didn't want her to be in pain. For the final six months of her life, pain control was all I had left to help her, other than prayers and words of comfort. This period was also difficult because, although I was showing care, she didn't always recognize it as such. Sometimes my help was just a nuisance to her, and she was so unsettled and hesitant to talk about the inevitable.

Dealing with the end of your wife's life is incredibly difficult because you know that your partner, your lover, your wife and best friend is going to be leaving and you can't change it. So I just concentrated on trying to make her comfortable. We did, though, seem to develop some patterns. I would get her a cheese danish from a local bakery every morning, a fish sandwich from McDonalds for lunch, and kept her in supply of Hershey's chocolate. It may sound funny, but that's what she liked to eat, and I wanted to make her comfortable. It reminded me of when she was pregnant and had cravings.

I think what helped my wife emotionally and spiritually more than anything else in her final days was having talks with our pastor. She would come by the house and talk to my wife frequently, and because they were both women, my wife began to open up and talk about her death a little bit. So our pastor helped my wife more than she knows. She read scripture to my wife, sang, and had a prayer just moments before she died. There was also a hospice nurse who had a huge impact in this way. I could hear them talking about "letting go." My wife seemed to have this funny idea in her head that she was letting everyone down by dying. This frustrated her and our family, because it wasn't the case.

The week before my wife died, we had a wonderful day outside. I was able to put her in the wheelchair, and we took a walk around the neighborhood. But she was getting weak and didn't want to go back in the house. And when I took her inside, she was upset.

Of course, when my wife died that was a rough day. The funeral was helpful, and I still go to the cemetery about once a month. I sit on the headstone opposite the grave. I actually feel at peace and recharged after I go. I take care of the plot. This is important to me, and sometimes my five-year-old grandson goes with me. He often asks to "go see Grandma's grave."

I'm not sure I have any advice for men in this situation other than to say, do the best you can and try to come to grips with the reality. Just keep caring. Use the family and people around you, like hospice, to give you the support and strength you will need to take care of your wife during her last days.

~Emory

Five Things to Remember:

- Allow your wife to tell you what she needs, and respond with that care.

- Make your wife as comfortable as possible.

- If you are facing an end-of-life journey with your wife, don't hesitate to call hospice.

- Remember, this may be more difficult for you than for your wife.

- Be present.

Chapter Eleven
The Next Chapter

Perhaps nothing is more welcome after breast cancer than a return to normal or, to put it another way, a new chapter. This next chapter, for you and your wife, will hopefully include a fulfillment of your dreams, whether that includes burning your mortgage, seeing your children married, spending time with grandchildren, or even traveling to those distant, exotic locations. You can look forward to these things and so much more.

In time, your wife may come to regard herself as a "breast cancer survivor." Or she may go months at a time without ever thinking about breast cancer (or the mastectomy or chemo, for example). She may become involved in breast cancer organizations or participate in a breast cancer walk ... or she may not have a desire for these at all. Likewise, you may discover that your new "normal" is much like before. Time has passed, and the memory of the breast cancer journey you took with your wife seems more and more distant, even less clear, and you may forget certain discussions or decisions that were made. Perhaps the breast cancer journey itself no longer defines what the two of you have become or where you are going. It's just something that happened.

Regardless of how you live this next chapter of your life, there are some bits and pieces of the breast cancer experience that may hang on to some couples for the duration. This is not true for all, mind you, but there are always those women who must live with certain side effects.

This is by no means an exhaustive list, but the following represents the most common post-cancer experiences for women—and also for men.

Chemo Changes

Doctors have known for some time that chemotherapy can sometimes have long-lasting side effects. Again, this is not true in every case, and these side effects vary by person and intensity and description, but chemo does affect some women. One phrase that I recall hearing to describe this experience is "chemo brain."

This phrase may be overly descriptive, however, as what this implies is that, somehow the brain has been altered by chemotherapy. Such is not the case. Rather, what is being described is a variety of symptoms that some women exhibit. For example, some women describe having "hot flashes." These momentary rises in temperature (whether real or imagined) can leave women feeling that their bodies are ovens, or that suddenly they are sweating for no apparent reason. Some women—particularly older—describe these as being similar to menopause.

Doctors are, of course, uncertain about the realities of these side effects. Some maintain that the symptoms are psychosomatic or could be related to the stress and anxiety of worrying about cancer.

But regardless, some women do affirm that these feelings are real and that they must take measures to cope. Over time, most of these symptoms fade, but in the years immediately following these major traumas on the body, these chemo flashes can be more pronounced for some.

Another symptom is forgetfulness. Again, not by any means a universal experience, but some women report that they are unable to think as clearly following chemo, or may simply have moments when they forget details or events they would normally retain. Some of this may be attributed to the natural aging process, but younger women report similar experiences, too.

Many doctors have noted that chemo has been known to hasten the onset of menopause. Many of the symptoms may have just as much to do with menopause as the chemo itself, and that is why some women look to hormone replacement therapy. If your wife is on the cusp of menopause before taking chemo, be aware of the fast-track changes that might be coming her way—and yours.

Husbands can help with the post-chemo chapter by being aware of the times, places and situations that might throw their wives into these sudden changes. They can also help by gently reminding their wives of important events, or reminding their wives to do more writing and recording on paper. A little urging never hurt anyone, and with a bit of gentle assistance, most women who experience these symptoms will eventually return to their "old" selves.

Exercise and Diet

Most women, post-cancer, do make changes to their lifestyles. For example, some women will make a point to eat a healthier diet, and they may bring home stacks of cookbooks and recipes that will give them a new direction with their cooking. Men can play a large role in supporting this by being agreeable to these dietary changes.

Men who, for example, got into the habit of being a food guru pre-surgery might actually enjoy seeing it through to the other side. All of those fresh fruits and vegetables, the frozen casseroles, the bottled water—these things can be part of the new chapter. A little carryover from the former life is a great thing.

Other women will want to make changes to their exercise regimen. This, in fact, was one of the biggest changes my wife made—and continues to make. Many women discover a newfound joy of exercise post-cancer. Whether it be walking, hiking, or riding a bicycle, many women find a new appreciation for staying active. Others might want to take up master gardening classes or ballroom dancing. But no matter what it might be, be certain that you encourage your wife to explore her active side. Even if she shows only a hint of promise, give her accolades and, wherever possible, participate with her.

Soon after my wife's recovery, we decided to take up wine appreciation. We began travelling to wineries (and sometimes hiking to them), and this has been one of our greatest joys for the past decade. We've not only learned a great deal about wine and winemaking, but we have started writing a book together and have also added photography to that mix. All things considered, this single interest has combined diet, exercise and our common interest. Not only have we explored wineries in Napa Valley, and Washington and Oregon states, but we have made wide-sweeping forays into Michigan and other points around the Midwest. We have a lot more to learn, but this pursuit has kept us in shape, made us healthier, and given us reason to travel together.

Another up-and-coming exercise therapy is yoga—specifically, stretch yoga classes designed specifically for breast cancer survivors. These classes, which combine low-impact exercise, stretching, balance and meditation, are now very popular. Many women and their husbands are discovering the benefits of this method. Yoga allows women to continue their stretching routines—exercises they may have learned post-surgery—and carry it forward into whole-body therapy.

In the years ahead, don't overlook those things that can change your life. Find a passion that can keep you both active and engaged as you move into this new chapter.

Career Changes

I would be remiss if I didn't mention career as one potential chapter in your new life. As noted earlier in this book, many women have such a powerful experience with breast cancer that they feel compelled to make major life changes afterward. Sometimes a career can be a part of this. But your career might change, too.

In fact, statistically most people will change careers several times in their lives. It is a rare thing indeed to find someone who works in the same career (and certainly for the same company) for a lifetime. Today, not only are companies more likely to terminate, but employees are far more likely to move on to greener opportunities.

Post breast cancer, you may also discover you have the itch to make a change. Even for a husband, this is not uncommon. Sometimes being a caregiver awakens other aspects of a person's psyche and heart to pursue other dreams. Perhaps you feel you are in a dead-end job, or maybe you've been feeling you are in a rut. Other men can feel undervalued or underappreciated.

I'm not saying a career change is inevitable, but if you are feeling an urge to change, grow, or expand your repertoire of gifts or intellect, it might be helpful to at least explore your options. And if you do, I'd highly recommend that you seek a career counselor in your area. A good career counselor can give you a gifts-assessment test that can identify areas of interest or other career choices you might not have considered before. No counselor will tell you to leave your job, but receiving this feedback can be some of the most stimulating conversation. The counselor may also affirm that you are in the perfect career and give you some accolades or pointers that will inspire you and set you on a new path inside your current career.

In this new chapter of your life, don't neglect working on *you* after you've had the opportunity to help your wife.

What About Lymphedema?

If your wife did have lymph nodes removed or had a follow-up surgery in the node area, the physicians no doubt explained there is a chance of lymphedema. This is a medical term that describes the painful swelling of the arm caused by fluid buildup in the tissues. Perhaps you have seen some women who wear a sleeve during these flare-ups, or your wife may have friends who have suffered from this.

Of course, not all women develop lymphedema, and there are certainly some precautions your wife can take to help alleviate the risk or to cope with the side effects. Sometimes the psychological impact of lymphedema can be just as, if not more, painful as the physical condition itself. Many women with this condition (or when they have a flare up) will retreat and not feel comfortable going out in public. This is probably more of an issue with her than it is with you, but she may feel that others are looking at her or wondering why one of her arms is swollen or reddish.

While I was writing this book, I did ask some women to describe what lymphedema feels like and how they react to it. Some described the condition as a "full" feeling in the arm, while others said it was more of a burning sensation. Some just described lymphedema as painful. Some women noted that when they had a flare-up of the condition, they simply placed their arm in an elastic sleeve, took medication, and went about their business as usual. Others did confess they felt more self-conscious during these times and were less likely to venture to the store or participate in some public event. Some said the condition made them feel tired, and they simply needed to focus on getting better until the condition passed.

So the symptoms and after-effects of lymphedema can vary among women. Moreover, some women develop the condition soon after surgery, while for others the condition may come on some years later, and for many women, not at all.

If your wife does have lymphedema, you may also experience a certain amount of anxiety about it. Some men may not want to press their wives when the condition flares up; other men retreat from the condition and may not want to spend time with their wives when she is hurting. Lymphedema, however, does not mean a woman can't enjoy her usual pursuits or that she must be treated differently.

But women with lymphedema can use help. If your wife has this condition, or you fear she may develop the condition later in life, there are several things you can do to help stave off the onset or help her cope with the condition. Among the most helpful points would be:

- Remind your wife to drink plenty of water (the recommended six to eight glasses a day). Hydration seems to play a key role in alleviating lymphedema and its symptoms.

- To the point listed above, encourage your wife to exercise. This means keeping her arms in shape—toned and strong. Lymphedema is exacerbated in fatty tissue. So the firmer and fitter her arms are, the better. Don't shy away from using light weights.

- Don't allow your wife to lift heavy objects, however. Don't allow her to overexert herself or stress the arms and shoulders too directly.

- If you are flying, remind your wife to wear loose-fitting sleeves. Air pressure differences can cause tissues to fill with fluid, and flying is known to make lymphedema more painful.

- When flying, drink even more water.

- If your wife is accustomed to carrying her purse or a bag over the at-risk arm, remind her to switch to the other side. Again, this is just a point of stress, and it is best to allow the at-risk side to remain unburdened.

- Create a care package for your wife that she can carry with her or keep in the car. This pack can contain some ointment, perhaps some antibacterial cream, an elastic sleeve to fit and some aloe. This kit can give her peace of mind and can come in handy if she does have an unexpected flare-up.

- Keep her supplied in some of her favorite hand and body lotions.

- Some women also swear by acupuncture for relief from lymphedema. The medical community certainly has mixed opinions about acupuncture. It is one of the many alternative therapies not officially recognized by the American Medical Association. If your wife does suffer from lymphedema, however, she might talk to other women who have used acupuncture for relief.

As you can see, lymphedema, when it does occur, is one of those constant reminders of breast cancer. It is a chapter of your wife's post-cancer experience I hope she does not have to face. But if she does develop the condition, now you know how to help. You've been through much together, and this will be another step.

Although this is one of those ongoing chapters, you'll be facing it in the same way you've faced all of the other hurdles. You'll do it together. And you'll certainly have a newfound appreciation for the phrase, "It's a good day."

Reclaiming Your Life

As you already know, breast cancer is not so much an ending as a beginning. Once you have stretched beyond the years when breast cancer is a daily specter, you can begin to reclaim some of the pieces of the life you left behind. You might begin to take longer vacations or find that you have more time to pursue favorite hobbies or recreation, or you may even work longer hours in your career.

Eventually you will begin to embrace new ventures, and you and your wife will begin dreaming new dreams. Some of the old fears will dissipate, and you will find that your wife will actually be encouraging some of *your* pursuits! When you get there, give yourself a pat on the back. Time itself doesn't really heal wounds. People heal wounds. And you were integral to your wife's recovery from breast cancer.

Well done!

Final Thoughts

My hope is that this book has offered both substance and practicality. Here you may have found more than you wanted to know about many aspects of breast cancer and not enough when it comes to your specific questions. But I do hope you won't allow this book to be your one and only source of information.

There is a wealth of knowledge and experience out there, and in the final pages of this book you can find a detailed bibliography that can lead you to other superb books, as well as a guide to breast cancer organizations and other resources—all of which can benefit you and your wife.

And don't forget to take advantage of your own doctors and specialists, as well as the friendships you have made through this experience. There are always people willing to talk and to listen. And these are often the most important resources we have.

May your journey together be filled with love, life and laughter.

ഇറ

First Person

I had always had a fear that my wife would develop lymphedema after she had several nodes removed under her left arm. These symptoms didn't show themselves until a year after the surgery.

We were on vacation in Florida at the time, and my wife noticed one afternoon that her arm was getting red. We assumed it was from too much sun, and neither of us thought much about it. But later that night my wife was experiencing some rather severe pain. That's when we started talking about lymphedema and trying to remember everything the doctor had told us.

I was able to do an Internet search the next morning, and I brought back a lot of information to my wife. She was sort of a basket case. I kept trying to reassure her that we could deal with the symptoms, and we began taking steps to help her manage. The flight back home was uncomfortable for her, but once we got settled into our old routines and started doing more research on methods and treatments, she was able to control a lot of the symptoms when she felt them coming on.

She bought one of those restriction sleeves, and that really helped. She also checked her diet and started drinking a lot more water. I think all of these things helped her. Or at least she claims they did. Well, her pain wasn't as severe in most cases.

The main thing with my wife was that she was so self-conscious about it all. She had a tendency to withdraw during the episodes, and sometimes she got depressed. I had to play cheerleader a lot, you know ... help drag her out of the house and keep a life.

We've both done much better coping with lymphedema than we thought we would at first. It's not something we think a lot about now. It's been eight years since the first flare-up, and it's kind of old hat now. Some days are worse than others, of course, but she doesn't want it to keep her from doing the things she enjoys. I admire her for that. I really do.

I don't know. Maybe I've helped, too. It's not something you want to happen, but when it does, you just have to cope with it and find new ways to manage. It can be done. And men just need to ask other guys about it. Some women have remarkable ideas that can help those who suffer from lymphedema, but you have to ask about it.

Anyway, that's what I've learned. I'm just glad the cancer didn't beat us.

~Rick

Five Things to Remember

- Many women experience a desire to make changes following breast cancer (you may, too).

- Chemo can have adverse and life-altering impacts on the mind and body, so be prepared to recognize what some of these changes are.

- Work every day to encourage your wife and build her self-esteem post-cancer.

- If your wife develops lymphedema, there are many ways you can help manage her symptoms and her pain.

- Approach each day with the philosophy that the "best is yet to come."

Appendix of Terminology

For a more complete understanding of any medical terms, please consult a medical dictionary or a physician. Throughout this book, certain terms have been used, and this appendix is meant to be a thumbnail guide to this terminology. This is by no means comprehensive, and if there are other questions you have about a phrase or medical term, please ask your doctor to explain more fully.

એજી

Androgen: a male sex hormone, sometimes used to treat breast cancer.

Alopecia: baldness. Many women at some stage of chemotherapy may lose their hair. There are wigs and head coverings women can use during this stage.

Axilla: referring to the armpit area.

Benign: noncancerous; no evidence of cancer

Bilateral: meaning both sides of the body. In reference to breasts, it can mean there is a tumor in each breast or that a mastectomy or surgery is needed on both breasts.

Biopsy: the procedure of removing a tissue sample to determine if cancer is present in the body or that area of the body. A biopsy is the most common way that doctors determine the presence of cancer and its general location.

Blood count: a test to measure the number of red and white cells in a blood sample.

Breast cancer: technically a cancer inside the breast tissue or breast ducts, and is highly treatable. Breast cancer can be fatal, however, if the cells grow rapidly or if the tumor spreads to other parts of the body.

Breast prosthesis: instead of a breast implant, some women will opt to wear a silicone or fiber-filled implant inside the bra.

Breast self-exam: a procedure for examining the breast thoroughly once a month in order to check for the evidence of suspicious lumps. These exams should normally be performed at the same time each month and are suggested for all women after puberty.

Cellulitis: an infection occurring in soft tissues. As far as breast cancer, certain tissues are at a greater risk for cellulitis following the removal of lymph nodes. This can be accompanied by pain, swelling and warm sensations.

Calcifications: these are the small calcium deposits in the breast, most commonly in the milk ducts, which are discovered during a mammography.

Cancer: a tumor or cellular structure that divides and reproduces abnormally and can spread through the body.

CAT scan or **CT scan**: an x-ray view of the body in sections.

Carcinogen: any substance that initiates or promotes the development of cancer. Cigarette smoke and asbestos, for example, or known carcinogens.

Chemotherapy: the drug treatments or injections designed to rid the body of cancerous cells.

Clear margins: a margin is an area around a cancer cell or tumor which is free from cancer. In breast cancer terminology, this refers to the area of breast that is surgically removed. Sometimes, if the physical feels that all margins are clear around the tumorous tissue, there will be no need for further radiation or chemotherapy.

Clinical trials: some women may choose to become part of a study either during or after their procedures. Doctors use these clinical trials to learn more about breast cancer and effective treatments.

Cohort study: any study of a group of people who have something in common. Studies are usually conducted over a period of time to see what happens to these people when subjected to other treatments or medications.

Diagnosis: the process of identifying a disease through description of characteristic symptoms and testing. With cancer, an early diagnosis is preferred to a later diagnosis.

Duct: referring to the ducts of the breast through which milk can travel to the nipple.

Estrogen: the female sex hormone produced by the ovaries.

Genetic: relating to genes or inherited characteristics.

Grade: often used as another name for "stage," but here referring to the size and type of cancer. The lower the grade, the smaller the cancer and the earlier the stage.

Homeopathy: a system of therapy using small doses of certain drugs that can produce symptoms similar to those in diseased people. One belief is that homeopathy supports the immune system.

Hormone therapy: a cancer treatment that removes, adds or blocks hormones.

Hyperplasia: an abnormal growth of benign cells.

In situ: this means cancer is confined to the point of origin or "where it sits." In breast cancer terminology, that means the cancer or precancerous cells are confined to the milk ducts.

Invasive breast cancer: cancer that has spread from the milk ducts and glands to other parts of the breast or the body.

Latissimus flap: flap of skin and muscle which is taken from the back to complete reconstructive surgery on the breast in lieu of implants.

Lobules: the glands in the woman's breast that produce milk.

Lump: a mass (cancerous or benign) that has been found in the body.

Lumpectomy: a surgical procedure where a smaller amount of tissue is removed (with clear margins) around the tumor or cancerous region. This is in lieu of a full or partial mastectomy.

Lymph node: the immune system glands that filter cell waste.

Lymphedema: a swelling with fluids in the arms or legs. The removal of lymph nodes and radiation treatment can place a patient at risk for this condition, which usually manifests itself on the side of the body where the breast/nodes were removed.

Mammary glands: the breast glands that produce and carry milk.

Malignant: cancerous.

Mastectomy: surgical removal of the breast tissue.

Metastasis: The spread of cancer cells to other parts of the body.

Mitosis: cell division.

Needle biopsy: biopsy with a needle.

Negative: a good thing in medical terminology—meaning that no cancer was found.

Observational study: a study in which a factor is observed in a group of people.

Oncologist: a medical specialist trained to detect and treat cancer.

Pathologist: a medical specialist who determines if a tumor is benign or cancerous and who assigns the grade to cancer.

Pectoralis major: the muscle underneath the breast.

Phlebitis: irritation of a vein.

Platelet: a cell formed by bone marrow that is necessary for clotting in the blood. Platelet transfusions are sometimes used in cancer patients to control bleeding.

Port: a small device placed under the skin through which medicine can be administered.

Positive: in medical terminology this means cancer has been detected in the body.

Primary site: the place where the cancer begins.

Prognosis: an expected outcome; the future prospect for a patient.

Prosthesis: an artificial limb, or in the case of breast cancer, a breast prosthesis which is usually attached inside the bra.

Rad: in radiology terms, a dose of absorbed radiation.

Radiologist: a medical specialist who reads mammograms and can perform needle biopsies.

Reconstruction: the rebuilding of the breast post-surgery either with tissues from the patient's body or with implants.

Rectus abdominus: stomach muscle.

Recurrence: meaning cancer that comes back or returns.

Remission: usually referring to the disappearance of cancer in the body and sometimes to cancer-related symptoms.

Risk factors: anything that increases an individual's chance of getting a disease. As far as breast cancer is concerned, some risk factors include an immediate relative who has had breast cancer, a high-fat diet, smoking, etc. Breast cancer specialists can provide a more extensive list of these factors.

Risk reduction: techniques used to decrease the chances of getting a disease. In breast cancer, these might include quitting smoking or reducing fat in the diet.

Silicone: a synthetic material used in breast implants and known for its resiliency, pliability and durability.

Stage: in reference to breast cancer, it refers to the size and advancement of the cancer.

Surgical oncologist: a breast surgeon who removes cancerous tissue from the breast.

Tamoxifen: a common hormonal therapy.

Tumor: a mass or lump (benign or cancerous).

Helpful Web Sites

There are literally thousands of Web sites devoted to breast cancer. While the list below is by no means exhaustive, it does represent some of the best known or, in my estimation, most helpful places to begin. Some of these sites are informational. Others are inspirational. Still other sites offer support networks and advice to families or even end-of-life help. A wider search will no doubt produce some favorites of your own, but these are great places to begin.

℘ℭ

American Board of Medical Specialists (www.abms.org): Provides information about physician qualifications and ratings.

American Cancer Society (www.cancer.org): Largest national society for all cancer-related information.

Bald is Beautiful (www.baldisbeautiful.org): Dedicated to helping women through hair loss associated with chemo.

Cancer and Careers (www.cancerandcareers.com): A marvelous site devoted to helping women balance cancer and career.

Cancer Information Service of the National Cancer Institute (www.nci.nih.gov): Basic information service on cancer.

Cancer Information Service of the Canadian Cancer Society (www.cancer.ca): Canadian information provider on all cancer-related topics.

Cancer Care Inc. (www.cancercare.org): Free professional support to cancer patients and their families.

Caring Bridge (www.caringbridge.org): Provides free Web site and support services to those who need inspiration and prayers of family and friends.

Dr. Susan Love (www.drsusanloveresearchfoundation.org): Web site of Dr. Susan Love, a trusted name in breast cancer information.

Living Beyond Breast Cancer (www.lbbc.org): Wonderful support site containing information about recovery and post-surgery/treatment factors.

Mamm (www.mamm.com): National organization and magazine devoted to all things breast-related.

Men Against Breast Cancer (www.menagainstbreastcancer.org): A help line where men can post questions and answers to breast cancer-related topics.

National Cancer Survivors Day Foundation (www.ncsdf.org): Information on the annual celebratory event for cancer survivors.

National Center for Complementary and Alternative Medicine (www.nccam.nih.gov): For those seeking therapy and recovery options.

National Coalition for Cancer Survivorship (www.cansearch.org): Helpful site for cancer survivors.

National Hospice Organization (www.nhpco.org): The best end-of-life organization to assist patients and families.

National Lymphedema Network (www.lymphnet.org):Super help site and support network for women affected by lymphedema.

Susan G. Komen Foundation (www.komen.org): National organization for breast cancer fundraising, research and annual walks to support these endeavors.

SHARE (www.sharecancersupport.org): Survivor-led support for women and their families.

Stand by Her (www.standbyher.org): Men's help site.

Y-Me National Breast Cancer Organization (www.y-me.org): Premier research and information center.

Young Women United Against Breast Cancer (www.youngsurvival.org): Premier website for younger women affected by breast cancer.

Other Resources

There are many magazines and other material devoted to the breast cancer experience or support team. As noted elsewhere in this book, here are some of the best places to begin.

Care Notes (www.onecaringplace.com)

Cure Magazine (www.curetoday.com)

Mamm Magazine (www.mamm.com)

Outcalt, Todd: *Caring Through Cancer* (CD)—may be ordered at www.toddoutcalt.blogspot.com.

Bibliography

Altman, Roberta and Sarg, Michael. *The Cancer Dictionary* (Facts on File, 1992)

Anderson, John. *Stand By Her* (AMACOM, 2010)

Braddock, Susan. *Straight Talk About Breast Cancer* (Addicus Books, 1996)

Dackman, Linda. *Up Front: Sex and the Post-Mastectomy Woman* (Viking, 1990)

Eiler, Larry. *When the Woman You Love Has Breast Cancer* (Queen Bee Publishing, 1994)

Fore, Robert M.D. *Survivor's Guide to Breast Cancer* (Smyth & Helwys Publishers, 1998)

Gross, Amy. *Women Talk About Breast Surgery* (Clarkson Potter, 1990)

Hirshaut, Yashar & Pressman, Peter. *Breast Cancer: The Complete Guide* (Bantam, 1997)

Lange, Vladimir. *A Survivor: Your Guide to Breast Cancer Treatment* (Lange, 1998)

LaTour, Kathy. *The Breast Cancer Companion* (William Morrow & Co., 1994)

Link, John. *The Breast Cancer Survivor Manual* (Owl Books, 2000)

Love, Susan. *Dr. Susan Love's Breast Book* (Perseus Publishing)

Murcia, Andy. *Man to Man: When the Woman You Love Has Breast Cancer* (St. Martin's, 1990)

Outcalt, Todd. *The Healing Touch* (HCI Books, 2005)

Parkinson, Carolyn. *My Mommy Has Cancer* (Coping Books)

Silver, Marc. *Breast Cancer Husband: How to Help Your Wife (and Yourself) Through Diagnosis, Treatment, and Beyond* (Rodale, 2004)

Sokol, Bruce. *Breast Cancer: A Husband's Story* (Crane Hill Publishing, 1997)

Index

About the Author

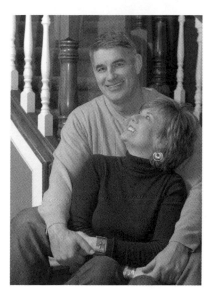

Todd Outcalt is the author of thirty books in six languages including *The Healing Touch* (HCI), *Candles in the Dark* (John Wiley & Sons), and *The Best Things in Life Are Free* (HCI). He has written widely about breast cancer, and his work has been featured in such magazines as *Cure, American Fitness*, and *The Way of Saint Francis*. Todd is a United Methodist pastor of thirty years who has helped hundreds of families through cancer, and he lives with his wife, Becky, in Brownsburg, Indiana where they enjoy hiking, kayaking, and travel.